PROUDLY PUBLISHED BY SNOWBOOKS

COPYRIGHT © 2006, 2017 IAN OLIVER

SNOWBOOKS LTD
INFO@SNOWBOOKS.COM
WWW.SNOWBOOKS.COM

BRITISH LIBRARY CATALOGUING IN
PUBLICATION DATA.
A CATALOGUE RECORD FOR THIS BOOK IS AVAILABLE FROM THE
BRITISH LIBRARY.

PAPERBACK
ISBN 978-1-911390-36-7

THIS NEW EDITION PUBLISHED OCTOBER 2017

IAN OLIVER
BOXING
FITNESS

A GUIDE TO GET FIGHTING FIT

NEW EDITION

FIRST THINGS FIRST
FOREWORD & ACKNOWLEDGEMENTS

Boxing Fitness as a book was not my original intention, or invention, but came about when my friend and colleague Wayne Rowlands showed Snowbooks' editor Emma Barnes the bulging folder of notes I had amassed while working at The Academy Gym in Hoxton Square. Emma convinced me it would make a handy guidebook for beginners, or people who simply wanted to get fit through boxing training, having wearied of other exercise routines.

One reviewer on Amazon complained my style as "too chatty", a criticism I wholeheartedly endorse – my intention was to give the impression I was telling you what I recommended in an informal manner, as I would at the gym, not like a drill sergeant.This is definitely NOT intended as a text book, just somebody advising you how to train.

The book is quite obviously aimed at beginners, no seasoned, accomplished fighters will learn anything new here; they are not my intended audience.

People I trained in this method always seemed to enjoy the freshness of a new regime, which was always my wish.

As I first wrote the book in 2006, I felt it was time for an update, and I wanted to add the section on pad-holding from "Punch Your Way to Fitness".

I hope the new, enlarged and, hopefully, improved version will help the reader achieve a new improved version of their personal fitness.

ACKNOWLEDGEMENTS

Kind thanks to my colleague Victoria Mose from the YMCA training and development department for ensuring the accuracy of the advice that follows.

Also to my good friend Savash Mustafa (Doctor of Osteopathy) for his kind assurance that the training regimes contained within are not life threatening.

Grateful acknowledgements must also go to Emma Barnes, Pete Drinkell and my good friend and colleague Wayne Rowlands who made this book a reality instead of a possibility; and to Sally and Cheryl, whose constant moaning forced my hand.

Respect and special thanks go out to Bob Breen, Terry Barnett, Gordon McAdam and Alex Turnbull, from all of whose motivational classes I borrowed so heavily, and still continue to do so.

A WORD OF WARNING...

It almost goes without saying that a book on boxing training will involve some vigorous and demanding physical effort. If you have any concerns about your health then I must stress the importance of getting clearance from your doctor. If you have not participated in any training before, or not for some time, then start gradually, always taking the easier options and limiting the training times. Too many people have the impression that if exercise doesn't hurt then it is not achieving anything: this is not the case. You should, and my fervent hope is that you will, enjoy your exercise. Never forget that you have the rest of your life to get fit.

CONTENTS

CONTENTS

FIRST THINGS FIRST
INTRODUCTION

The majority of people who read this are not interested in boxing as a profession, or even as a competitive amateur; those people started out as kids, or at least teenagers. Late starters who became world champions, such as Rocky Marciano and Sonny Liston, in their twenties, are very few and far between. Successful competitors have usually been taught, often from a young age, by seasoned trainers who know how to get them battle-hardened, while keeping them within the confines of a particular weight.

This book is mainly for those people who want to get fit using boxing training as a conduit, as opposed to simply using weight training, aerobics, running or other activities that they feel have lost their stimulus as stand-alone exercises. Participants have never failed to surprise me. In the past I have trained actors, dancers, doormen, executives, painters, sculptors, musicians, lawyers, DJs and professional sportspeople among the growing band of devotees to boxing training.

In my experience there are a few fundamental reasons why people turn to boxing.

- They want something new in the way of training that will be demanding but refreshing. No matter how placid and controlled people are by nature most of them can derive great satisfaction from hitting something hard. Taking your frustration out on a punchbag is a wonderful form of psychological self-help. Buy a punchbag and skip going to an analyst; what better form of anger management can there be? Cheaper too, even with gym membership.

- They fancy a shot at "white collar" boxing competition, in what was once, traditionally, a blue collar sport. Schools dropped boxing from their sports program as it was considered decadent, archaic and politically incorrect. A new program of boxing in schools has now had a widespread and enthusiastic reception. It is of a non-contact variety with the emphasis on getting fit and combating child obesity. In the digital age of the computer and 'gaming' the results will be interesting.

○ Boxing still thrives in the armed forces and many universities, but boxing clubs need a large membership to generate sufficient revenue if they are to pay the rent; rising rents have put paid to many of the old established clubs.

○ They are not looking to get a huge build, but seek the lithe muscular look that fighters develop, as opposed to bodybuilders. Despite the claims of many other fighting/martial arts, boxing is still seen as the most popular form of self-defence. You get two-for-one on this score as you become able to fight, and in condition to do so as well.

○ As part of an introduction to integrated or mixed martial arts such as Muay Thai, Panantukan, Kickboxing, Vale Tudo and Jeet Kune Do.

Boxing has become marginalised in the media as a minority sport, coverage is usually reduced to major or controversial contests, usually involving heavyweights. Some broadsheets sports pages neglect fight coverage completely. The resurgence has come from the public interest in doing it as opposed to merely watching it. A few years ago the shiny, hi-tech gyms would never have included a punchbag among their glittering array of machines and equipment, in full view of their yoga and pilates classes, but clients wanted them, and they wanted to know how to hit a bag, and how to skip rope like a fighter. New gyms are often stocked with an array of punchbags and even boxing rings. Films about boxing remain popular; Million Dollar Baby and The Fighter garnered major awards and critical acclaim, and people still dab their eyes as they watch The Champ.

I have included sections on exercise that supplements boxing, such as running, core fitness and weight training; I must point out that in these sections I have aimed at the specific training in relation to boxing, as obviously, I am unconcerned with marathon running or bodybuilding. More detailed and extensive training in all these excellent disciplines can be found in "helpful literature."

THE BENEFITS OF BOXING

Boxing training will improve strength, speed, aerobic and anaerobic fitness, balance, agility and muscular and cardiovascular endurance, as well as providing a basic means of self-defence.

In closing, the following quotes are common in what can be referred to as 'gym maxims', it is just a case of dissecting the bad – "no pain – no gain" (erroneous), and "go hard or go home" (macho drivel), from the good "USE IT OR LOSE IT". Trust me – this is the one that holds true.

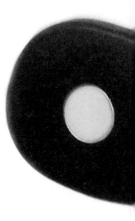

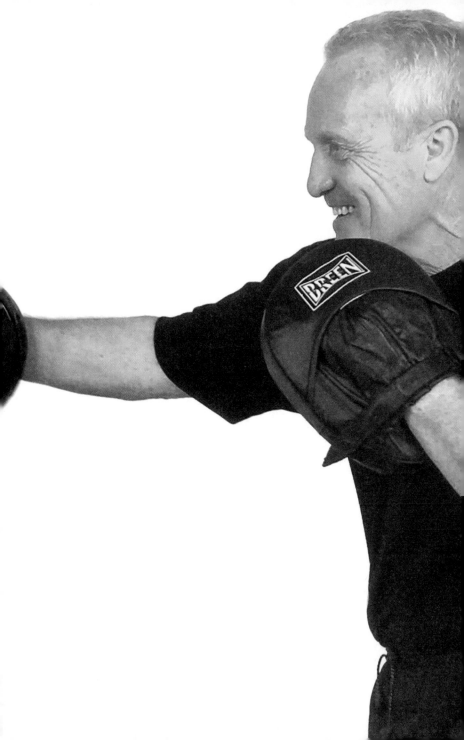

TECHNIQUE

At this opening stage I apologise to all left-handed practitioners (known as "southpaws" in boxing parlance). Transpose left and right instructions and all should be fine. Whether you are right-handed, left-handed or ambidextrous – the basic technique is the same.

It must be stressed that you can only learn a certain amount about boxing from a book, just in the way a book cannot teach you to ride a bike, face a fast bowler or sink a ten-foot putt; you need the physical component. If later you become serious about your boxing you may want to join a club; many clubs realize you may only want to train, not spar or compete, and if you pay a membership or entry fee, they are usually fine with that. The best way to locate a boxing club is an online search (BBC run a 'find your local boxing club' page). Type in "find a boxing club". Clubs or gyms specializing in Mixed Martial Arts will usually have sessions dedicated to boxing. Many of the large chain gyms – Virgin, Fitness First and others – provide boxing facilities such as bags, focus pads and even a reasonably-sized ring in some cases.

I would advise going to watch proceeding at two or three clubs before making your choice. Look for somewhere that takes training seriously but is nevertheless friendly, if you do not want it to be like a Royal Marine induction course.

GETTING STARTED

I start with the crucial aspect of the stance, as if you are not standing properly at the very beginning then nothing is going to fall in place. The renowned trainer Charlie Goldman, who transformed an awkward Rocky into a legendary heavyweight champion was, some years after Marciano had retired undefeated, recruited to work with Tom McNeely, an opponent of the then reigning heavyweight champion, Floyd Patterson. Even an alert and astute trainer as Goldman despaired of his charge, stating he "couldn't even get him to stand right."

Patterson won by a 4th round knockout, after flooring his opponent ten times.

Charley Goldman was frequently quoted, and his last words are reputed to be "Only suckers get hit by right hands."

THE STANCE

Imagine you are standing on a large clock face, your left foot on 12 o'clock and your right foot at twenty past twelve. You should try to maintain this stance for most of the time you are boxing, making sure you never cross your feet. Your bodyweight leans very minimally forward from the waist, in a manner such that you are not bolt upright, but very slightly crouched. Your chin should be low enough to retain a tennis ball underneath it, but your eyes are on the target. Both elbows are tucked comfortably against the ribs and the right hand, semi-closed and ready to block or hit, is close to the chin, so you can just see over the top of it. The left hand is held at the same height as the right, but forward of it, with roughly 12" between the gloves. The left glove is closed. The position of the hands is generally referred to as 'the guard'.

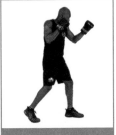

The stance

Novices will often shape up to lead with their strong hand, and are surprised to learn that they will need to lead with their less competent hand, unless they have the massive good fortune of being ambidextrous, in which case they can take

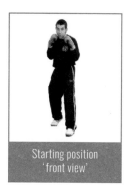

Starting position
'front view'

their pick. It should be explained why they are required to adopt this stance, rather than simply expect them to take it on blind faith. There are three basic reasons in my opinion.

○ The more competent dexterity of the right hand will provide a better defence to your face than the left, so needs to be the rear hand.

○ The rear hand delivers the big punch, but it needs the lead hand to act as a range finder (or, colloquially, the 'can opener') to provide the opportunity to be unleashed. Leading with the more powerful hand and trying to deliver the power punch off the weaker side would be a futile exercise. The jab is typically the weaker punch, but enforcing sound technique, abetted by specific power training, can turn it into a formidable weapon.

○ Try moving around, in the manner described above, except with your right foot leading; it soon becomes apparent to most students that the rear foot is more dominant, more powerful and a more comfortable option for precise and controlled boxing footwork, in addition to providing a stable base. Get on the 'good' foot – station it at the rear.

Arms and legs both need to feel relaxed, and the knees should have a 'springy' feel. Remember – loose limbs travel faster – avoid tension at all costs.

HOW TO MOVE

All you need to remember when you first start is:

○ The front foot takes you forward

○ The back foot takes you backwards

○ If you want to move to the right, lead off with the right and push off with the left foot

○ If you want to move to the left, lead off with the left and push off with the right foot.

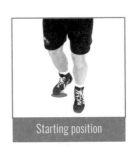

Starting position

It is as easy as it sounds.

Stay on the balls of the feet and practice maintaining good balance as you move around. Do not bounce; move in a sliding fashion, gliding like a ballroom dancer – a tough ballroom dancer.

○ Going forwards; step with the left and allow the right to slide after it, maintaining the '20 past 12' stance.

○ Going backwards; step back with the right foot and slide the left foot backwards to follow it. The 'slide' should follow the 'step' in rapid succession. Practice should very soon allow you to perfect this simple manoeuvre.

Bouncing around in a fashion somewhat akin to that of a boxing kangaroo is labour-intensive, impractical and not good to look at. (Glance in the mirror if you don't believe me.) Instead, move around in an energy-conserving, smooth, sliding motion.

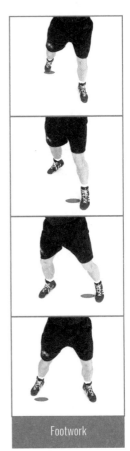

Footwork

BALANCE

Good balance is crucial, as poor balance will almost certainly result in poor performance. The correct stance, with arms and legs relaxed, and shoulders above the hips (not leaning too far forwards) will be a good base

7

to work from, but self-help involving core training to strengthen and develop the stabilising muscles can help enormously.

DIRECTION

Beginners invariably tend to circle to their left, which seems more natural to right handed people. Always moving left is a bad habit to get into, as a) it makes your movement predictable, and b) it brings you closer to the right-hand power punch of an orthodox boxer (but works favourably against a southpaw, wherein the left-hand becomes the power punch). The answer is to constantly circle in both directions, making yourself unpredictable, but mainly circling away from your opponent's 'big' hand. Don't just go forward and backward: lateral movement is important.

HOW TO HIT

MAKING A FIST

Many beginners are unsure of the way to make a 'fist' in the correct fashion to prevent damage to the hand, especially the thumb. Most injuries beginners incur are to the wrist, usually through failure to keep the arm straight when landing the punch, or to the thumb, due to incorrect positioning of the thumb on contact.

The 'major' knuckles (the large top row) are the only part of the hand you should make contact with. The rest of the bones of the hand are brittle, and easily damaged when meeting very hard objects, e.g. a heavy bag, a maize bag, a skull.

The following guide is for the benefit of the absolute novice.

- ° Settle the hand comfortably into the glove, pulling hard on the wristband to ensure a snug fit. When buying gloves, allow a little room in them for hand wraps (see "Hand wraps", overleaf). Your hand may expand slightly during training, so never buy tight-fitting gloves. It is advisable to own your own gloves. Some gyms have a "lucky dip" box whereby you can have the loan of a pair of what are usually sad, distressed and discarded gloves;

these invariably give off a less-than-fragrant bouquet, having been bestowed a legacy of perspiration from a few hundred hands.

○ Close the hand, leaving the thumb in the "thumbs up" position.

○ Draw the thumb tightly against the fingers.

HAND WRAPS

Anybody intending to work on punch bags or focus pads would be well advised to wrap their hands. For the princely sum of £3-£5 you can prevent hand and wrist injury and the likelihood of delayed pain quite easily. See chapter on "Equipment" for selecting your wraps, but I always advocate the 'elasticated' version, with a Velcro closing, which hold their shape and are less likely to become unravelled in use. Wraps are essential for beginners, some of whom tend to 'cock' their wrist, as opposed to maintaining a straight arm with a 'flat' wrist action on striking.

Hand wraps simplified (I hope).

There are various ways of wrapping, but for anybody who finds the diagram misleading, I'll run try to run through the stages.

1. Most good wraps have a Velcro closing. Make sure it is on the inside, but if you forget – twist it over to the right side before final fastening.

2. Hook the loop over your thumb (top left, overleaf).

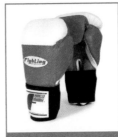

Competition gloves for amateur boxing. Only punches landed with the knuckle part of the glove (the white area) score points.

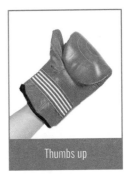

Thumbs up

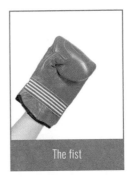

The fist

3. Take two turns around the wrist (top centre).

4. Take the wrap across the palm of the hand, between the third and fourth fingers, back around the wrist, then back across the palm to go between the index and middle fingers (2nd row on left).

5. Around the base of the thumb, and then between thumb and index finger (2nd row extreme right).

6. Back around the thumb, then between the 4th and 5th fingers.

7. From here on wrap around the hand with a small overlap each time (as with a bandage).

8. When the hand is fully wrapped (4th row extreme right) continue, with small overlaps, up to almost the middle of the forearm. By taking it as far as this helps to protect the wrist.

9. Finish should resemble photograph at bottom right.

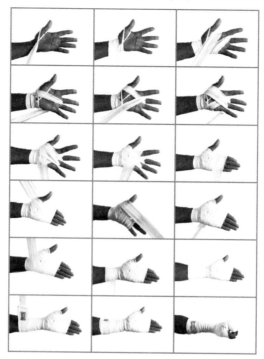

If this is all too confusing – slip the loop over your thumb, wrap your fingers to the first set of knuckles, then back again to the wrist, encircle the wrist and fasten off close to halfway up the forearm. Going between the fingers adds linear support to the hand, but as long as the hand is fully wrapped in a firm fashion and provides some padding, that should suffice to get you started. Most trainers will be happy to give instruction on this.

Most people tend to work out their own system of wrapping, and then stick with it. If you have enormous hands then you may want to add a second roll of tape; if you have concerns about injuring your hands you can lay some thin foam over your hand prior to wrapping it, keeping it in situ with surgical tape before applying your wraps. Applying surgical tape between the fingers, along the length and breadth of the hand on both sides will give added support.

THE PUNCHES

THE LEFT JAB

Both George Foreman and Joe Frazier always maintained that the jab was the most important punch in boxing, and it is the first punch the novice must master before moving on. It is the most dependable weapon for initiating an attack and is an effective form of defence when under pressure. It can be thrown from a safe, defensive stance, limiting the degree of risk taken; it can quite easily be 'doubled' or 'trebled' for added effect.

It is essential (as in all punches) to make firm contact with the knuckle part of the glove, ensuring only the large knuckles of the hand are employed.

The jab acts like a spear, thrust sharply towards the target. It should be snapped – never employed in a pawing action, which is a waste of time and energy. It should be delivered crisply and cleanly, and retracted instantly after contact is made. Take the shortest and most direct route to the target i.e. a straight line.

○ Push off powerfully from the rear foot (you must raise the heel) to ensure a transfer of weight forward, going

11

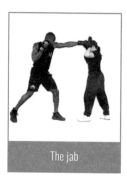

The jab

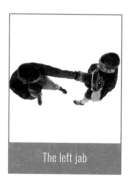

The left jab

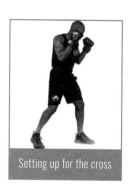

Setting up for the cross

from the 'passive' to the 'active' mode. Consider the ball of the rear foot to be the starting point, which will initiate the move: the small spark that starts a big fire.

○ Turn the hip in the direction of the punch-line, which will ensure the weight of the backside gets involved. 'Arm-only' punches are totally ineffective – learn to punch your weight by getting a good hip turn as you deliver the punch. Whether you are hitting a bag or a pad make it your intention not to merely punch 'to it', but to punch 'through it', which will give more power.

○ After you make contact you should retract the hand instantly, bringing it back along the same path it travelled out along, at the same time keeping your right hand in a defensive position alongside the jaw. Always keep both hands up – think defensively.

THE STRAIGHT RIGHT / RIGHT CROSS

The 'cross' is, strictly speaking, when the rear hand is fired over or under an incoming lead, 'crossing' the opponent's arm. It has become, in common parlance, to simply mean a 'straight right' (or left, in the case of left-handers). Using the term 'cross' makes it common to both 'orthodox' and 'southpaw' boxers. It always denotes a punch delivered by the rear hand.

○ This is where you can unleash the

beast, a highly satisfactory sensation, as you hit with your 'big' hand. Resist the temptation to swing wildly, or 'follow through', Rocky-style. Control is essential to sound technique. This needs to be a piston-like action, delivered dynamically from a solid base, followed through to its full extent, and, as with the jab, retracted instantly after being thrown, regardless of the effectiveness of the delivery. Again, as with the jab, it comes back along the path it travelled out along.

○ Drive off the ball of the rear foot; the more power you can muster will be reflected in the strength and speed of you punch. Speed cannot be underestimated; a slow, ponderous or lazy effort is hardly likely to prove effective. 'Snap' is an essential ingredient of all punches; it is the magic factor that allows a lightweight to throw a punch that is more effective than that thrown by some heavyweights, due to the shock value. Aim to 'make it snappy'.

○ This being a hard punch I make no apology for reiterating that you must ensure you make contact with the top row of knuckles, delivered with a slightly downward action to ensure the knuckle area alone makes solid contact. Turn the right hip and shoulder powerfully in the direction of the blow to ensure your full weight gets behind the punch. As this punch is of a higher risk tariff than the jab, you do not want to waste it.

○ Keep the shoulders over the hips. Don't stretch to reach the target. Move the whole body forward as a unit, taking a small step with the lead foot if necessary to ensure your backside (the heaviest unit of the body) is moving forward. Don't leave your power behind.

SHUT THAT DOOR!

Both the jab and the cross can be likened to the action of a slamming door. When throwing the jab, the right-side acts as a

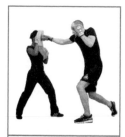

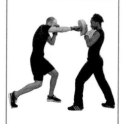

The right cross

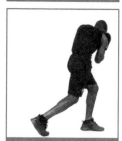

Setting up for left hook

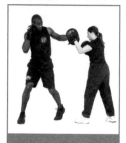

The hook

solid base, like the hinged side of the door, allowing the left side to slam forward.

When the forceful right-hand punch is thrown, the roles are reversed as the left side acts as a hinge while the right-side hammers to its target, hopefully akin to an outhouse door in a force nine gale. Allowing excess movement of the stabilising side interferes with the overall dynamic.

THE HOOK

The hook is usually a little harder for beginners to master, which is generally due to over-complication; it is a relatively simple punch to learn, best thrown in a natural fashion and not over-stylised, which can reduce effectiveness. The left hook is more commonly used than the right hook by right-handed boxers, by virtue of the fact it is nearer the target and thus arrives with less notice of its arrival than a right hook, which is thrown from further back. I apologise if this seems self-evident. Many people were under the (mistaken) impression Henry Cooper must be naturally left-handed, because he regularly packed such a tremendous left hook, like the one that floored Muhammad Ali. Anyone who wants to know what a perfect left hook looks like should watch footage of their encounter, and note the speed at which the hook was thrown and the flawless technique.

The left hook is used to mount a lateral attack and penetrate the defence of an opponent's protective right hand, or to counter against a right-hand punch by hitting over or under the right hand. The right hand is a natural follow-up to the left hook or as a body punch having avoided an incoming left jab.

Basic steps are:

- Shift your weight to the side you intend to launch the hook from, turning the hip and shoulder away slightly. Slide the back foot in a little so the feet are in a 'quarter past twelve' position, as the narrowed base will allow a more dynamic turn to create power, as well as making the manoeuvre simpler.

- The arm should be bent at the elbow (see variations below) at about 90 degrees. The other hand is pulled close to the head, on defensive duty.

Raise the left heel vigorously and pivot the left hip simultaneously and make a violent (no point in mincing words here) turn and slam the left hand against the target with the upper knuckles leading and the thumb (tucked in tight) on top as you make contact. The instant after making contact, or not, as the case may be, whip the hand back to the original defensive position.

VARIATIONS ON A HOOKING THEME

The shape of the arm will have much to do with the amount of power applied when throwing the hook.

- If the arm is bent at the elbow, to form a right angle, this will encourage a strong hip turn, which should result in greater punching power.

- If the arm is at an 'obtuse angle' – greater than a right angle – there will be reduced power, as there is less hip turn.

- When the arm is at an acute angle, with the fist closer to the body, a full forceful hip turn needs to be applied to register a punch with the arm in this position, but should result in an extremely potent blow at very close range.

For all three varieties, it is advisable to momentarily shift the feet into a 'quarter past twelve' stance immediately prior to delivery.

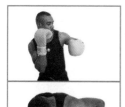

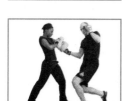

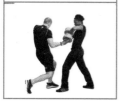

The Shovel Hook

The shovel hook is a short-range punch to be employed when in close proximity to an opponent; ignoring the anti-social aspect, think of it as 'fighting in a phone box'. The rear foot needs to slide forward into a 'quarter past twelve' position, making it easier to thrust the hips forward for maximum effect.

It is sometimes referred to as a 'body uppercut' and is, in effect, a modified version of the uppercut (see 'Uppercut', below), but with the arm being rammed forward at a 45-degree plane, as opposed to vertical, as in the uppercut. The non-hitting arm is held in a close defensive position to protect against a counter, as this is close-range contact. As with the hook (and the uppercut) it is essential to raise the heel.

This punch can be delivered with equal efficacy by either hand.

The Uppercut

In the photograph it can be seen that Corey makes preparation, prior to the explosive conclusion.

The uppercut is strictly a close-range punch, usually delivered with the stronger hand. The following relates to right uppercut.

Basic steps are:

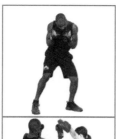

- ○ Feet should be, ideally, in a quarter past twelve stance.

- ○ Drop the right shoulder below the intended target area, then drive upwards in an explosive fashion with

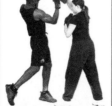

The uppercut

the hips as you punch upward in an almost vertical plane. A powerful push-off from the rear heel allows the hips to travel upwards forcefully. The true weight of the punch comes from below the belt – not the arms.

○ The defending hand is retained close to the head to guard against a counter punch.

○ The punch should not travel not much more than 12", or it will be 'telegraphed' – and easily avoided. After delivery, the hand must be returned to the guard position.

○ This punch is best developed on focus pads, but do not be tempted, after contacting the pad, to 'follow through' skyward, as this will leave your head unguarded: a bad habit to get into.

JABS AND CROSSES TO THE BODY

A slightly different technique is employed when throwing jabs and crosses to the body. The hitter should bend at the knees but not lean forward as this will result in a loss of power as well as increasing the risk of vulnerability to a counter. Try to keep the shoulders over the hips.

Jab to the Body

With the rear hand defending the head, bend the knees (never from the waist), keeping the shoulders over the hips, gathering momentum from the ball of the rear foot as the leading arm is speared at the target fully extended – using the full extent of your reach is important when making this shot. The left hip and shoulder should follow the direction of the punch; the arm is retracted instantly after throwing the punch.

The Cross/Straight Punch to the Body

As with the jab, bend at the knees, keeping the shoulders over the hips as much as possible, the left hand alongside the head for protection. Again, the power is drawn by driving forcefully off the ball of the rear foot, turning the right hip and shoulder

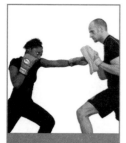

Left jab to the body

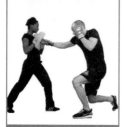

Straight right to the body

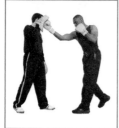

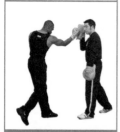

Right 'screwed' punch

along the path of the blow. Fully extend the arm for maximum effect.

Both above punches call for a rapid 'in and out' action. The bent knee position is not one to be caught in by a fast counter.

The 'Screwed' Punch

This punch is at its most effective when fired from the rear hand, straight from the chest, with the palm facing upward. Power is derived from a forceful drive of the hips and a dynamic push-off from the ball of the rear foot, as Owen demonstrates (bottom left). The idea when using this punch is usually to attempt to drive it between the defending gloves, using the element of surprise.

Feinting / 'Kidding'

When using all the above punches there is a customary ploy, essential to anybody considering progressing to sparring, that of 'feinting', also known as 'faking' or by the popular boxing term 'kidding' – the art of pretence. It is a technique used to mislead an opponent into thinking you are about to throw a punch. This is best practised on focus pads whereby you can attempt to dupe the pad-holder – preferable to taking your untried technique into a sparring session.

HOW TO DEFEND

If there is something more important than learning how to hit then that will be learning how not to be hit: the art of defence. In boxing an action begets a reaction and it is important to know which defensive action to take.

Always bear in mind that if you and an incoming punch are travelling in the same direction at the same time the impact is lessened enormously. If you are travelling in the opposite direction of an incoming punch, thereby in its direct path, the result can be the opposite – disastrous.

The best analogy is a car crash. A rear end shunt (you are moving away from the impact) can prove minimal, whereas a head-on collision is unthinkable. Hence the old term "roll with the punch."

DEFENCE AGAINST THE JAB

Can the jab really be a hard punch? After I saw the Jamaican light-middleweight Simon Brown knock out the defending champion Terry Norris of the U.S. with a jab I realised just how potent it can be in the hands of a great exponent, regardless of the fact Norris won the rematch.

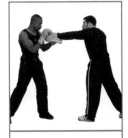

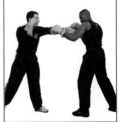

Defence against the jab

The lesson is – never underestimate the power of the jab.

Your rear hand should be near the jaw, making a small circular movement in readiness for action. Block the incoming jab with the semi-clenched rear glove, 'fielding' it to deflect it away from your head, not slapping it away as excessive travel by your rear hand could leave your head exposed to a follow up hook-off-the-jab shot. Wait until the jab has passed your own lead hand before getting involved – going out to meet the anticipated blow will leave a large gap – an incoming left hook sized gap if you are not careful.

In the photograph above Wayne, the pad holder, fires a jab with the focus pad which

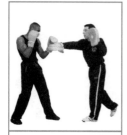

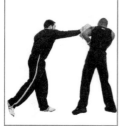

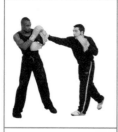

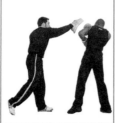

Defence against the
straight right

Owen defends with his rear hand with his chin down and eyes always on the opponent.

DEFENCE AGAINST THE CROSS

The lead hand, with which an opponent will jab with, is close to you and needs quick reactions. The rear hand is usually far enough back for you to get more notice of its approach. For this reason, your defence is three-fold.

○ Steer the incoming hand away with your lead hand, as depicted.

○ Turn your shoulder tucking your chin close to your chest to glance over your shoulder, your right hand in front of your face, your right arm tight to your body. The blow should land on your shoulder or shoulder blade and thus nullified if you pull back at the same time.

○ Simply step or sway backward to let the blow fall short of its target.

DEFENCE AGAINST THE HOOK TO THE HEAD

I have chosen three basic techniques (hopefully the most usable).

The Block

Raise the arm to block the blow, taking it on or around the elbow. This is the most reliable form of defence against close range hooks. The left hook might well be considered the most dangerous punch to defend against as it comes around fast from out of the line of vision and subsequently is seen very late – too late for some people!

'Bob and Weave'

This is inadvisable against a much shorter opponent. As you become aware of the hook arriving, bend at the knees keeping your head and shoulders directly above your hips with your eyes on your opponent.

Do not bend forward excessively from the waist. Keep your hands and arms tucked in tight to the body, although a crisp shot to your opponent's body from the 'bob' position is the ideal bonus. Come up as the blow has sailed (hopefully) over your head, moving slightly to the side the punch came from – think of this move as 'down and out', whereby you bob down and weave out of the way.

Swayback / Snapback

This ploy works best for anybody who is facing a much shorter opponent. Simply sway (or snap) backwards to avoid the swing of the arm and be ready to sway back again to a more vertical stance from where you can launch a counter attack.

In the photos depicting the defences both

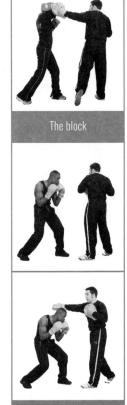

The block

'Bob and Weave'

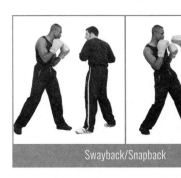

Swayback/Snapback

21

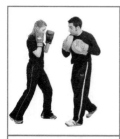

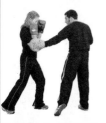

Defence against
body shots

left and right attacking hooks are shown. These defences; the block, bob and weave, and swayback work against both left and right hooks.

DEFENCE AGAINST BODY SHOTS

The general defence to employ against most body attacks is to move backwards or sideways in the same direction as the punch arrives, thereby avoiding or lessening impact. Use your arms held closely in front of your body in order for your upper arm and elbows to nullify any impression on your body.

With body hooks, ensure your elbows are tucked in tightly against your ribs in order to absorb a lateral attack. Ensure you are moving away from the impact at the same time for efficient damage limitation.

(See "Boxing Drills" – glove under arm drill).

'SLIPPING'

Using lateral movement to avoid an incoming punch is referred to as 'slipping', pulling the head off line by reacting sharply while if possible throwing a counter punch. This technique requires a great deal of practice to gain confidence in attempting it, particularly as the margin of error can be slender. Pad work is essential prior to going on to try this in a sparring session.

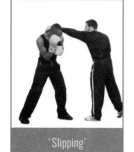

'Slipping'

MOVING THE HEAD

It may seem glaringly obvious that to avoid being hit in the head you will need to move it. Don't wait for a punch to come before moving it – get in the habit of moving it constantly – a moving target is hard to hit. Your opponent, even with your glove buried in his face, still has a pretty accurate idea of where you head will be – at the other end of your arm. The answer is to move your head and shoulders every time you throw a punch or feint to throw a punch. Simply move from the waist, shifting the head and shoulders in small, smooth movements. As with the moving target being hard to hit, keep your head and shoulders moving and hopefully you will be hard to hit. When you graduate to sparring try to employ a technique of ducking and bobbing with the head in small movements, in readiness for avoidance and to make accuracy difficult for your opponent.

SHADOW BOXING

Now you know how to move and how to hit and defend, you now have the opportunity to simulate these elements with some shadow boxing.

This is good exercise on its own and gives you the chance to rehearse the footwork and practise throwing all the punches. Only throw punches at your imaginary target when you stop moving – hitting on the move is best left to the legends such as Muhammad Ali. Don't put too much effort or power into your punches and try to stay totally relaxed throughout. Don't extend your arms fully or lock your elbows out. Try to keep in the '20 past 12' foot position as you cruise around. There is no need to wear your gloves as (hopefully) you won't be hitting anything. If you can find a partner to move around with you this will give a realistic sense of purpose to your efforts (referred to as out-of-range sparring), keep enough distance between you and your partner, about 5-6 feet, to prevent accidental and painful knuckle bumping (or worse).

Shadow boxing is an excellent warm-up, especially prior to sparring, but is suitable for warming up for most forms of exercise specific to boxing.

(See "Training with a Partner" chapter.)

SPARRING BASICS

The objective of sparring is to improve your combative skills in both attacking and defending. For the novice this is the moment of truth. Understand from the very start that if you go in for sparring you are going to be hit. Maybe not hit hard, but you will almost certainly will be hit and should learn to deal with it.

Not being hit, however, should be your primary objective. At a good gym sparring will be supervised by the trainer, who should make constructive points to the boxers, if only at the end of each round.

There are many basic tactics to employ and rules to remember. Here are a few of the more obvious points:

○ Chin down, mouth closed, eyes up.

○ Keep your eyes on your opponent at all times, never look away, and just in case nobody mentions it – defend yourself at all times.

○ Don't drop your hands, try to keep them on the same plane.

○ Don't cross your feet.

○ Move on the balls of your feet.

○ Always warm up before sparring – don't get 'caught cold'.

○ Taller opponents? Get close to take away their power. Long arms are less effective at close range as they need more leverage.

○ Shorter opponents? Use your reach advantage to keep them at bay. Do not let them get inside where their shorter arms can attack the body to good effect.

○ When under pressure – jab your way out.

- Circle in both directions, don't just be a linear boxer who only goes to and fro.

- Always move your head, in small movements.

- Feint to your opponent constantly, never stand stock still.

- Always ensure you know where you are in the space you are sparring in – do not get 'cornered' or 'cut off'.

- Never get angry as it will only lead to tension. Stay calm and relaxed.

- Feel tired/exhausted? Resolve to put in more roadwork in future.

- Don't worry about missing with punches. Even professionals can sometimes go a round only landing a few punches while missing with a lot. Regardless of this – be busy, throw a lot of punches if you can. Attack is a good means of defence, and can help to keep your opponent off-balance.

- Mix it up, don't just be a 'head-hunter'. Vary the attack to head and body.

- Don't spurn the chance to spar with somebody who is better, or more experienced than you – this is the best way to learn something.

- Orthodox boxer v. southpaw – mainly circle to your left, away from his left,

- Southpaw v. orthodox, mainly circle right, away from his right.

- Enjoy your sparring. It is one of the hardest and most demanding forms of training there is, even in short sessions.

BOXING TRAINING
BAGWORK

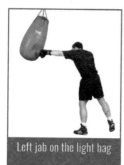

Left jab on the light bag

The punches covered in 'How to Hit' can be used on punch bags and focus pads, but I would advise beginners to start out on punch bags and preferably the light bag on their fledgling efforts, prior to graduating to the more densely-packed bags.

According to how well the gym you train in is equipped, you will usually have a choice of punch bags. My advice is to wrap your hands when working on the bag (see hand-wrapping in the "Technique" chapter) and wear good quality leather bag mitts. If your hands are a little sensitive or problematic in any way, you may prefer to wear 14oz sparring gloves to provide more cushioning. Hitting with bare knuckles may look macho, but could put you on the road to arthritic hands in older life.

There are a variety of bags, all beneficial to your training, albeit in different ways.

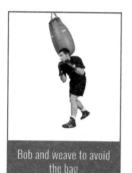

Bob and weave to avoid the bag

THE LIGHT BAG

Used for fast-punching combinations, it will have a generous swing which encourages changing your angle to avoid the bag as it swings towards you, and hit it while it is still 'on the move'. Do not put your hands out to steady it between hits; try to control it as you would an opponent, thereby making the training more functional. This is a great bag for novices to start out on.

You might like to try fast-hitting for 2 minute rounds, with a 30-60 second break in between. Try using 'bob and weave' as shown to avoid the swinging bag.

THE HEAVY BAG

Build up your punching power with hard, deliberate hitting on this bag. Striking the bag as it swings towards you will help to strengthen the power of your punch. It must be stressed that on hitting, the arm must be straight when throwing jabs and crosses, always making contact with the knuckle part of the glove. A cocked wrist can easily result in injury when using the heavy bag. This bag must be punched correctly, sloppy technique will result in pain or even damage to hand or wrist.

Mix up long and close-range punches. Don't just pound the bag aimlessly: try using combinations.

FLOOR TO CEILING BALL

An inflated ball suspended from above and below by springy but strong elastic cord. Every strike sends the ball veering off at an unpredictable angle, calling for improved accuracy as well as reactionary and timing skills. It also tests defensive skills, failure to move the head after hitting can lead to the ball hurtling back at a rate of knots which can surprise an unwary exponent. It simulates the movement of an extremely elusive moving target, very much akin to the way an opponent would move the head to evade punches. Be warned – I once witnessed a 'knockdown' inflicted on

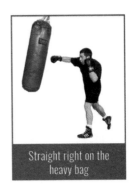

Straight right on the heavy bag

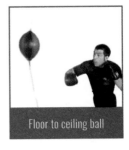

Floor to ceiling ball

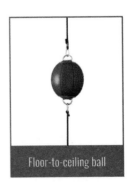

Floor-to-ceiling ball

a careless user – keep your head moving all the time. Don't try to land heavy punches, this bag calls for quick sharp punches.

This ball can make you look and feel foolish initially, as it is hard to fathom its movement and you are going to miss with a lot of your efforts, but it teaches valuable lessons in accuracy, timing and movement, and is worth persevering with.

TEARDROP BAG

Useful to improve hooks, shovel hooks, and uppercuts. Like the light bag it will swing to and fro and should be controlled by stopping it dead with a crisp punch – not a hug.

(See opposite page.)

SPEEDBALL

A small teardrop-shaped ball with a wooden platform mounted above. Good for improving hand speed, as well as arm and shoulder endurance as you have to keep both hands punching continuously. Drawbacks are that the punches are made in an unrealistic 'chopping and rolling', percussive fashion, and the staccato noise they make is incredible – you will hear it before you see it if somebody is using it. It benefits hand-eye coordination but may take a little while until you properly get the hang of it.

MAIZE BAG

Extremely dense and unresponsive piece of equipment, ideal for big punchers and potential big punchers, but better suited to experienced hitters and not much fun for beginners. Whether you are experienced or not, the hands should be wrapped for use on this bag – incorrect hitting could be injurious.

MAIZE BALL

Smaller version of the above, but as it is also filled with maize, so just as dense.

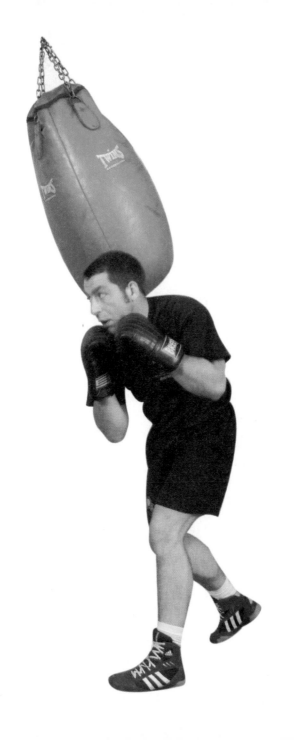

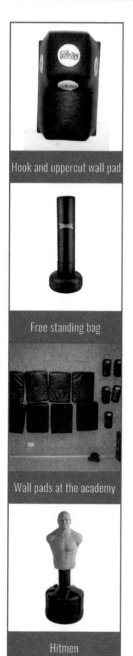

Hook and uppercut wall pad

Free standing bag

Wall pads at the academy

Hitmen

Suspended from above this item is useful for a 'hit and slip' drill; get your punch off, then 'slip' the ball as it swings towards you.

HOOK AND UPPERCUT WALL PAD

There is very little feedback from this static pad, which provides excellent opportunities to improve hook and uppercut skills. Straight punches can also be included in combinations.

PEANUT/ ANGLE BAG/ DOUBLE END BAG

A versatile hanging bag, usually referred to as a peanut bag simply because of its shape, lends itself to just about every punch you can throw at it. Try for 2 minute rounds in which you can use all your punches.

STANDBALL

An old favourite of boxing gyms but now something of an endangered species as they either have a base equivalent to the weight of an anvil, or need to be bolted to the floor – anything less and the whole thing topples over sideways. They are great for teaching novices straight punches and the junior versions are ideal for youngsters.

FREE-STANDING BAG

Tall and well-padded in the better made versions, this is a sturdy piece of equipment which is static but allows the user a 360 degree movement around it. They are popular in gyms as they can be tipped over and wheeled away and brought out when required. They need no fixings, but the supporting floor will need to be substantial as the large base needs to be filled with sand or water for stability, making it extremely weighty.

Try 2 minute rounds with 30-60 seconds' rest in between.

WALL PADS (IMPROVISATION)

In the photograph opposite, a collection of kick-shields have been hung from hooks to allow four people to train side-by-side simultaneously.

I saw a film of Cuban boxers training furiously on these bags, and although it is only suitable for straight punches it is great for allowing several people to work at the same time, punching at varying heights.

ANGLE BAG

Wide at the top with a functional taper allowing for uppercuts, body hooks, and shovel hooks, this is an extremely solid and useful bag. The top of the bag is a generous size for all your straight punches as well as head hooks. I declare this to be my favourite – the crown prince of punch bags.

'HITMEN'

This cheerless, unsmiling male Venus de Milo-type character is known, or at least marketed, as "Bob". He is one of several "hitmen" who have been used for target practice over the last few years, and his facial expression implies he is all too aware of what is heading his way. "Bob" seems to have outlasted his competitors in this vein of human-style punch targets but he has some serious deficiencies I am afraid. Apart from the fact he costs a small fortune, he also weighs a ton and is not durable enough for gyms (the one at our gym couldn't take the punches and he was soon decapitated).

PUNCH BAGS | INSTALLATION & COST

HOME (OR PRIVATE GYM) INSTALLATION

Most of the punch bags listed earlier are available for sale if you want to install one at home. There are, however, some aspects of home installation that must be taken into consideration. While you may not need a surveyor or architect, the advice of somebody in the building industry could prove invaluable.

If the bag is to hang in a garage, brick-built shed, barn, loft, or converted factory or school space, all it will most likely require is a stout hook from an ironmonger with the possible addition of a swivel hook. Some bags are sold replete with chains and an S-hook, while other come with merely a set of D-rings set in fabric, leaving you to source your own chains and hooks.

Regardless of fittings I would always recommend buying a punch bag that has been filled by the supplier rather than one you have to fill yourself – home punch bag filling enjoys about as much success as home dentistry, in my experience.

If your bag needs to hang from a wall, as opposed to hanging from a solid beam (at least 4 x 2), it will require a bracket, which vary in price according to their strength, density and quality of manufacture. At the time of writing they vary from around £18 – £65. The density of the brick wall should also be considered, because although the wall might be comfortably able to take the weight of the bag prior to use, the torque applied by heavy punching will place it under considerable stress. I have seen a bag, bracket and bricks all come crashing down together during a heavy training session because the installer did not realise the bricks were too soft when fixing up the bracket. When mounting on an outside wall it is sometimes necessary to insert a threaded length of steel running through to the outside surface, and secure both inside and outside with locking nuts and washers.

You may need to add some extras, possibly chains, carabiners/snap lock hooks for ease of hanging and taking down your bag, perhaps something more solid than s-hooks. A combined swivel and carabiner fitting should ensure smooth movement of the bag (selling at around £6 at time of writing).

ANCHORING YOUR BAG

You may want to tether your bag to the floor to limit how much it swings, or to anchor a floor-to-ceiling ball. At the time of writing this floor hook costs £8.

NOISE

Your efforts on the punch bag will resonate far and wide, as will the percussive beat of a speedball, which could almost be audible in the next postcode. If you have close neighbours they are unlikely to be sympathetic with your training methods.

FITTING

If fitting is impractical or would mean going to the expense of employing a professional, you may plump for a stand-alone bag. The only problem here is the weight as the base is filled with sand or water to prevent them toppling over or scooting across the floor. A concrete or strong wooden floor will be fine, but in the case of an upstairs room or flat it would be wise to first check out the strength and age of the floorboards.

STORAGE

Before you decide to hang a punch bag or install a stand-alone bag, remember that this beast is unlikely to be portable and your nearest and dearest may very possibly not warm to the appearance of it if it remains in plain sight – a possible reason why so many appear on eBay and the local ads.

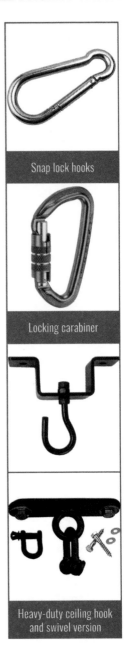

Snap lock hooks

Locking carabiner

Heavy-duty ceiling hook and swivel version

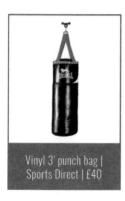

Vinyl 3' punch bag | Sports Direct | £40

COST

Punch bags can be reasonably inexpensive, a new vinyl bag, which is fine for home use, can cost around £40, whereas a top of the range full-size leather bag can cost anything from £100 to £350.

D.I.Y

(We are talking budget training here.)

While it will not square up to a pricey Reyes or Lonsdale leather bag you can nonetheless assemble your own punch bag, especially if it is as a temporary measure. I used to have an old army kitbag stuffed with rags (which took ages to work into a uniform shape) and hung over a beam with nylon rope, that served my purpose until I could afford a decent (second-hand) bag. I would recommend using a kitbag, hessian sack, laundry bag or similar to youngsters or anybody who is looking for a cheap and cheerful option for training.

Do not be tempted to use sawdust, a mistake some people make – even Mike Tyson in his pomp would not have enjoyed this dense, unforgiving medium very much. If hung in a damp shed or garage it doesn't take long to take on the consistency of wet sand.

Tear rags into strips, not in bundles, and if this still proves too hard on your hands, try mixing the rags with ripped-up chunks of foam rubber. If the bag swings too much try an inch or two of sand at the bottom of the bag – always remember to never to hit the bag at the bottom.

TIMERS

Whether you are working out on the punch bag or the focus pads, a timer is invaluable. You are likely to want to know when your 2 or 3 minute 'round' is over. Relying on a watch while wearing gloves or focus pads is impractical. Glancing up at a clock may be OK, but a timer with a clearly audible bleep will be perfect.

If the environment is not too noisy then the stopwatch on a mobile phone, iPad or a sports watch will be adequate.

See chapter 11, on equipment, for full timer details.

FOCUS PADS

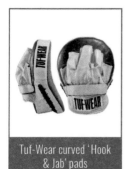

Tuf-Wear curved 'Hook & Jab' pads

Not many people are instructed in the correct procedure for pad holding; after a few aches and strains later they may well wish they had been. The following text hopes to advise you on how to hold pads without injury and at the same time provide maximum benefit to the person you will be holding the pads for.

PREVENTING PAINS & STRAINS

Learning to hold the pads properly is important for the prevention of elbow ligament injuries such as the dreaded 'tennis elbow', which affects the common extensor tendon of the elbow (top of the forearm). Its partner-in-crime 'golfer's elbow' (underneath the forearm) affects the common flexor tendon. Both injuries can be incurred without ever lifting a tennis racquet or a golf club; both are equally painful and debilitating. The injuries usually occur where the holder is too tense or simply has poor technique, which intensifies heavy punches, sending shock waves down the arm. Holding a pad rigidly while somebody is repeatedly smashing punches into it is a recipe for disaster. A correct and relaxed approach should eliminate any risk of this kind.

To prevent strains and overuse injuries the following specific stretches should precede a session of pad holding (see picture).

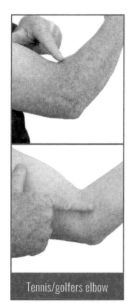

Tennis/golfers elbow

These stretches should be followed with wrist circling and finger shaking to get the wrists and hands loosened up.

PREPARATION

Simply holding the pads can be, per the intensity of the exercise, a workout. It is crucial that the person who is going to hit the pads should warm up properly and the holder should not be 'caught cold' either. The following warm-ups are tailored to the exercise which is to follow, as any warm up should be.

° Skip rope for 3 minutes.

° Shadow box for 2 minutes.

Bruce Lee used to throw 500 punches as part of his warm-up; why not take it a little easier on yourself and throw just 50 punches in a relaxed shadow boxing fashion as part of your pre-activity rehearsal. Once this becomes disdainfully easy, graduate to 100, or possibly more.

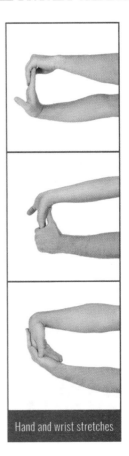

Hand and wrist stretches

HOLDING THE PADS

Pads usually come in two varieties, flat or curved. Both are fine but my personal preference is for the curved variety as I like the hand to be in 'cupped' shape as if ready to catch, as opposed to the hand being perfectly flat. This I regard to be a minor point.

The arms should stay relaxed to alleviate the 'shock' factor as mentioned above. The holder must learn to anticipate punches and absorb the energy in a technique similar

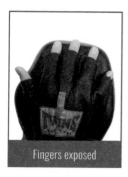

Fingers exposed

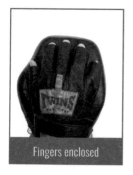

Fingers enclosed

to fielding a cricket ball or baseball, by allowing a little 'give' on contact, although without weakening the hitter's target area – do not over-retract the pad, they could hurt their elbow.

Some pads need to be carefully adjusted before use to ensure they fit snugly, whether the fastenings are Velcro or buckles. Floppy pads should be avoided and loose straps should be securely re-fastened or cropped to prevent the risk of eye injury. A flick in the eyeball from a whip-like length of leather may lead to injury and would certainly put a crimp in your workout.

If you have large hands or long fingers you will require pads large enough to accommodate the full length of your fingers or of an enclosed type. Squeezing your hands into pads that are too small can leave your fingers exposed to injury. A finger that extends to the very upper limit of the pad can quite easily be struck on the tip (see picture); as the rest of the finger is trapped in the pad this can prove very painful. Beginners cannot be expected to always land clean, accurate punches on the centre of the pad with unerring regularity, and the errant shot could be the one that hammers the fingertip hard enough to dislocate it. Pads that totally encase the fingers (not open-ended) are available.

Initially novice punchers should merely be encouraged to use sound technique, but with advancement should come 'counters' by the pad holder to remind the hitter to defend themselves always, exhorting them to keep their hands up and to move their head. A playful slap from a cushioned pad can warn of the dangers that may lie ahead from a sparring or competition glove. This action could be referred to as being 'cruel to be kind', although this tactic is inadvisable against beginners who may not initially be able to deal emotionally with this approach. In every case a clear warning of a likelihood of some contact during the session should be given (or you may never see them again).

Without constant reminders and reinforcement of good habits, the individual may as well work out on the bag.

HITTING THE PADS

Much simpler to explain – see the pad, hit the pad – what could be easier? It is good practice, however, to imagine driving your glove not just to reach the pad but as if you were hitting right through it. This should result in hitting a little harder and more likelihood of making contact when employed in 'the real thing'. Always think "eyes up, chin down".

CORRECT HOLDING

(Sorry, left-handers, please transpose instructions.)

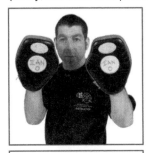

JAB/CROSS COMBINATION

Correct holding for jab/cross combination – note the pads are close enough to the head to imitate realism but not so close as to render the holder vulnerable to a "follow through" punch.

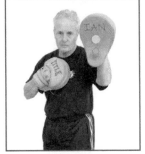

LEFT JAB TO HEAD

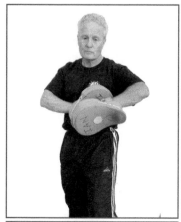

LEFT JAB TO BODY

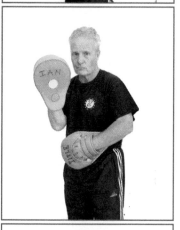

STRAIGHT RIGHT/
RIGHT CROSS TO HEAD

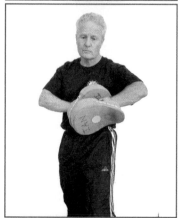

STRAIGHT RIGHT TO BODY

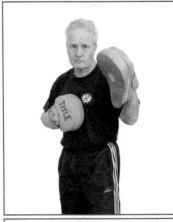

LEFT HOOK HIGH HEAD SHOT

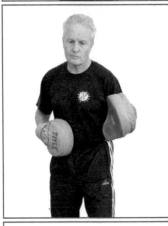

LEFT HOOK LOW BODY SHOT

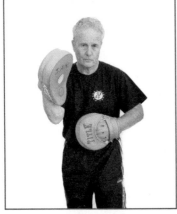

RIGHT HOOK HIGH HEAD SHOT

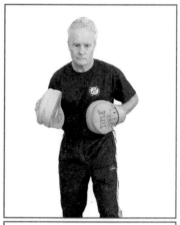

RIGHT HOOK LOW BODY SHOT

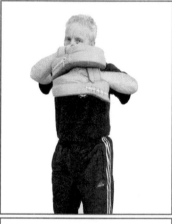

RIGHT UPPERCUT

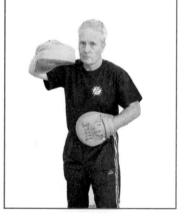

LEFT UPPERCUT

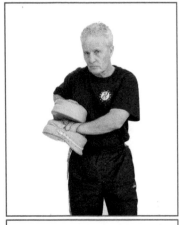

LEFT 'SHOVEL' HOOK

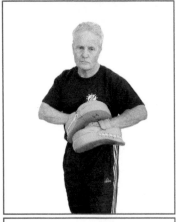

RIGHT 'SHOVEL' HOOK

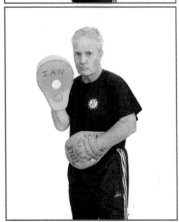

RIGHT 'SCREWED' PUNCH

Where a smaller/slighter person is holding the pads for a much more powerful opponent it may be advisable to employ the double pad holding technique (as shown).

43

IMPORTANT TIPS

○ Never hold for uppercuts with the pad directly under your chin (most people only get this wrong once).

○ When holding for novices do not hold the pads too close to your head as they will invariably lack pinpoint accuracy.

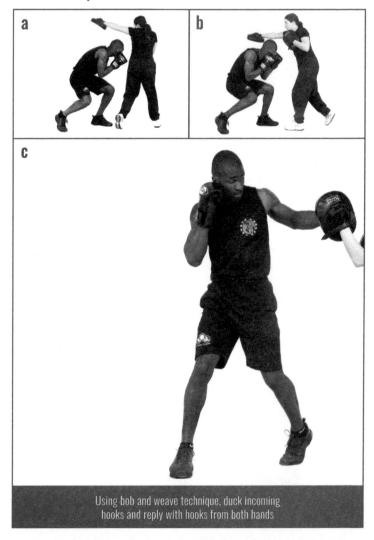

Using bob and weave technique, duck incoming
hooks and reply with hooks from both hands

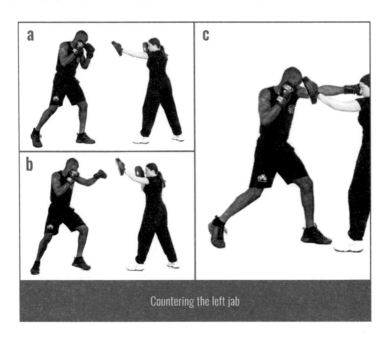

Countering the left jab

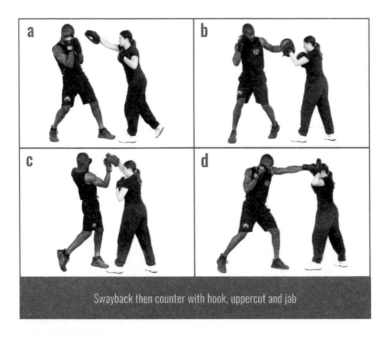

Swayback then counter with hook, uppercut and jab

45

COACHING MITTS

Coaching mitts introduce an advanced range of technique training, in particular that of a defensive nature.

These are a hybrid of sparring glove and focus pad. They consist of a huge, generously padded sparring glove with a focus area on the palm, which is strongly reinforced to sustain impact. They enable a coach to take training to the next level and introduce an element of sparring into the training regime. The trainee is now not only required to hit the target but to also defend against incoming punches thrown by a gloved hand (albeit an extremely well-padded one). It is an ideal precursor to actual sparring.

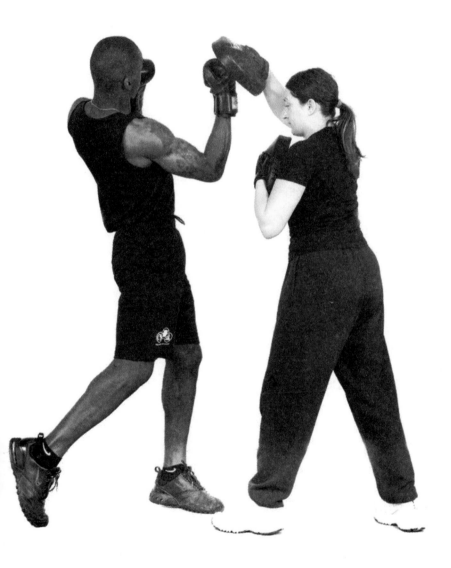

50 COMBINATIONS

In this section the punches are shown performed on focus pads, but exactly the same punch combinations can be used on punchbags.

It is fairly obvious that the increased demands of focus pad work renders it a more advanced form of training than merely hitting the bag, which is essential for both power and speed according to which bag is used. However, the pad training requires speed of thought and reaction as well as accuracy. Good quality training can be found on both.

1. MULTIPLE JABS

The very simplest combination is putting more than one jab together.

It is a useful manoeuvre, as the first jab can be deemed a 'range finder'.

The second and additional jabs should follow in rapid succession with no reduction in speed, power or correct technique.

2. JAB, CROSS

Regarded by many as "the old one, two", a stiff jab followed by a thumping right hand is a classic combination. Why throw the left first and not the right? The answer is that the right hand comes from further back, giving more time for avoidance – it needs the left to act a foil to set it up. It is essential to maintain maximum power, but also to ensure the left is retracted rapidly to protect the head the instant the right is thrown. The head must not be left undefended at any stage of the move.

3. LEFT JAB, RIGHT CROSS, LEFT HOOK, RIGHT HOOK

The jab and cross are thrown from a 'twenty past twelve' stance, but for the hooks the back foot may be slid forward to a 'quarter past twelve' stance, making it easier to turn the hip.

4. DOUBLE LEFT JAB, RIGHT CROSS, LEFT HOOK

5. LEFT HOOK TO THE BODY, LEFT HOOK TO THE HEAD, RIGHT UPPERCUT

6. LEFT JAB, RIGHT CROSS, LEFT HOOK TO THE HEAD, RIGHT UPPERCUT, LEFT HOOK TO THE HEAD

7. LEFT JAB, RIGHT CROSS, LEFT UPPERCUT, RIGHT UPPERCUT

8. LEFT JAB TO HEAD, STRAIGHT RIGHT TO BODY, LEFT HOOK TO HEAD, STRAIGHT RIGHT TO HEAD

9. LEFT HOOK TO HEAD, RIGHT HOOK TO BODY, LEFT HOOK TO BODY, RIGHT HOOK TO HEAD

10. JAB TO HEAD, JAB TO BODY, JAB TO HEAD, STRAIGHT RIGHT/CROSS

11. DOUBLE JAB COMING FORWARD, DOUBLE JAB BACKING UP FROM HOLDER

12. JABBING EITHER PAD, HIGH AND LOW, SINGLE AND DOUBLE

13. THROWING A 'HOOK OFF THE JAB' COMBINATION.

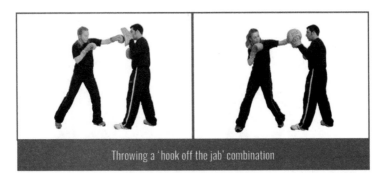

Throwing a 'hook off the jab' combination

14. HOOK OFF THE JAB, FOLLOWED BY STRAIGHT RIGHT/ CROSS, LEFT HOOK.

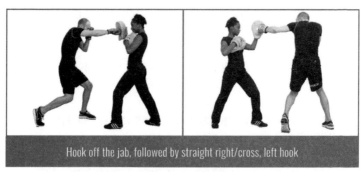

Hook off the jab, followed by straight right/cross, left hook

15. LEFT JAB, STRAIGHT RIGHT/CROSS, BOB AND WEAVE FROM HOOK THROWN BY HOLDER

Hooks can be thrown from both hands, according to which is executed more easily first.

16. BLOCK LEFT JAB THROWN BY HOLDER WHILE RESPONDING WITH OWN JAB

17. AS ABOVE, FOLLOW WITH STRAIGHT RIGHT/CROSS, LEFT HOOK

18. BLOCK INCOMING LEFT JAB, DEFLECT INCOMING STRAIGHT RIGHT, BOTH THROWN BY HOLDER, COUNTER WITH OWN LEFT JAB AND STRAIGHT RIGHT

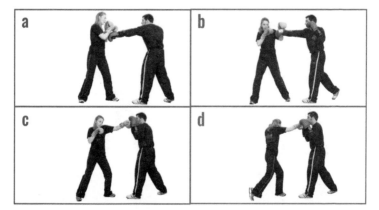

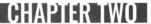
19. AS ABOVE, FOLLOWED BY LEFT HOOK, RIGHT HOOK

20. LEFT JAB, SCREWED RIGHT HAND, LEFT HOOK, RIGHT UPPERCUT.

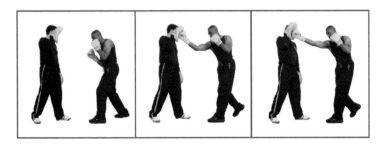

21. BLOCK LEFT AND RIGHT BODY HOOKS, COUNTER WITH HIGH/HEAD LEFT AND RIGHT HOOKS

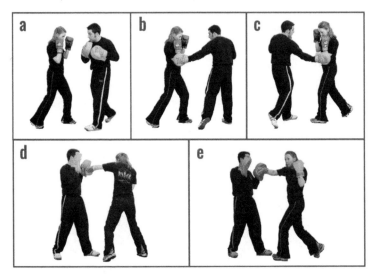

22. BLOCK LEFT AND RIGHT HEAD HOOKS, COUNTER WITH LEFT AND RIGHT BODY HOOKS

23. MOVE PAD AROUND FOR ALL PUNCHES

Providing a moving target increases the degree of difficulty. This is an advanced drill for the more experienced hitter, and the punches should be not thrown with full force for safety reasons.

24. SLAP & TURN

Initially the hitter faces away from the holder. Following a slap on the back, the hitter spins around, having to react to whatever punches the pads are held for. The position of the pads should be changed on each repetition.

25. HIDING THE PADS

Holder keeps the pads behind his back, then produces them smartly, giving the hitter only a brief time for rapid response.

26. 'SLIP' A LEFT JAB FROM THE HOLDER'S PAD BY STEPPING TO THE LEFT WHILE SIMULTANEOUSLY THROWING A RIGHT CROSS

Follow up with a left hook and a right uppercut.

27. HITTER DICTATES

The holder puts the pads up but does not know when the hitter will strike, or from which hand. This is a useful drill for learning to fake, by seeing if the hitter can dupe the holder.

28. DOUBLE JAB, RIGHT SHOVEL HOOK, LEFT AND RIGHT HOOKS

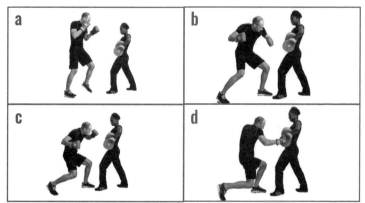

29. "FREESTYLE MODE"

Holder simply offers the pad, without verbal instruction, for the hitter to strike; with each pad offered the range of punches should include everything in the individual hitter's repertoire.

30. LEFT JAB, LEFT UPPERCUT, RIGHT CROSS, LEFT HOOK, RIGHT HOOK

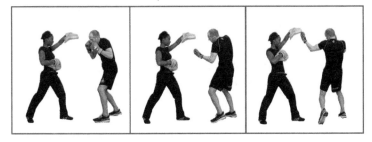

31. LEFT JAB, BOB AND WEAVE FROM HOOK, LEFT HOOK, RIGHT CROSS, LEFT HOOK

32. LEFT JAB, DOUBLE BOB AND WEAVE (FROM LEFT AND RIGHT HOOKS), RIGHT CROSS, LEFT HOOK, RIGHT CROSS

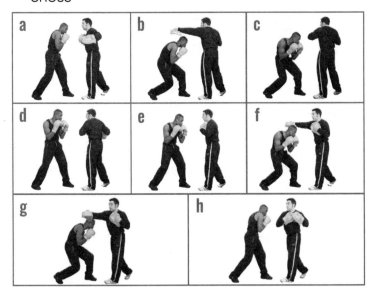

33. LEFT JAB, LEFT HOOK, LEFT HOOK, RIGHT CROSS

34. LEFT JAB, RIGHT CROSS, LEFT HOOK, RIGHT CROSS

35. LEFT JAB, LEFT UPPERCUT, RIGHT CROSS, RIGHT CROSS, LEFT HOOK, RIGHT CROSS

36. LEFT JAB, RIGHT UPPERCUT, LEFT HOOK, SLIP LEFT JAB, RIGHT CROSS

37. 'FAKE' WITH JAB BUT THROW RIGHT CROSS, LEFT HOOK, BOB AND WEAVE, LEFT HOOK, RIGHT CROSS, LEFT HOOK

38. LEFT HOOK, RIGHT CROSS, LEFT HOOK, DOUBLE BOB AND WEAVE (FROM 2 X HOOKS), LEFT HOOK, RIGHT CROSS, LEFT HOOK

39. DEFEND AGAINST LEFT HOOK, (COVER UP OR 'SNAP BACK'), LEFT HOOK, RIGHT CROSS, LEFT HOOK

40. DEFEND AGAINST LEFT HOOK (COVER UP OR 'SNAP BACK'), LEFT HOOK, BOB AND WEAVE, RIGHT CROSS, LEFT HOOK, RIGHT UPPERCUT.

41. DEFEND AGAINST RIGHT HOOK (COVER UP OR 'SNAP BACK'), LEFT HOOK, RIGHT CROSS, LEFT HOOK, RIGHT CROSS

42. DEFEND AGAINST RIGHT HOOK (COVER UP OR 'SNAP BACK'), RIGHT CROSS, BOB AND WEAVE, RIGHT CROSS, LEFT HOOK, RIGHT CROSS

43. LEFT JAB, RIGHT CROSS, DEFEND AGAINST RIGHT HOOK (COVER UP OR 'SNAP BACK'), RIGHT CROSS, LEFT HOOK, RIGHT HOOK

44. LEFT JAB, RIGHT CROSS, DEFEND AGAINST RIGHT HOOK (COVER UP OR 'SNAP BACK'), RIGHT CROSS, DOUBLE BOB AND WEAVE, LEFT HOOK, RIGHT CROSS, LEFT HOOK

45. LEFT JAB, RIGHT CROSS, LEFT HOOK, DEFEND AGAINST LEFT HOOK (COVER UP OR 'SNAP BACK'), LEFT HOOK, RIGHT CROSS, LEFT HOOK

46. 'FAKE' LEFT JAB, RIGHT CROSS, LEFT HOOK HEAD, LEFT HOOK BODY, BOB AND WEAVE, LEFT HOOK HEAD, RIGHT UPPERCUT

47. BLOCK LEFT JAB, BLOCK RIGHT HOOK RIGHT CROSS, BOB AND WEAVE, LEFT JAB, RIGHT CROSS TO BODY, LEFT HOOK, RIGHT CROSS TO HEAD

48. DOUBLE LEFT JAB, BOB AND WEAVE, LEFT JAB, LEFT UPPERCUT, RIGHT CROSS, LEFT HOOK, RIGHT CROSS

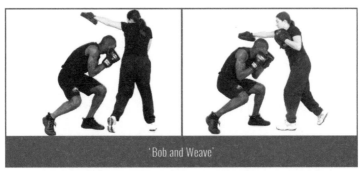

'Bob and Weave'

49. 'SLIP' LEFT JAB WHILE SIMULTANEOUSLY THROWING RIGHT CROSS, LEFT HOOK, BOB AND WEAVE, RIGHT SHOVEL HOOK, LEFT HOOK, RIGHT CROSS

50. LEFT JAB TO HEAD, RIGHT CROSS TO BODY, LEFT HOOK TO HEAD, LEFT HOOK TO BODY, LEFT HOOK TO HEAD, RIGHT UPPERCUT

SKIPPING

There are numerous reasons to make skipping part of your training regime (or 'jumping rope', for the benefit of any transatlantic readers).

- ° Boxing calls for upper and lower body synchronization, as does skipping, which improves upper and lower body co-ordination.

- ° Perfect for both aerobic (with oxygen) or anaerobic (without oxygen i.e. working flat out) training. It's your choice. Ideally you should use both systems alternately.

- ° Tones muscle and helps in fat reduction.

- ° Increases leg power and endurance.

- ° Improves agility and balance as upper and lower body must adapt to the harmony required for efficient skipping.

- ° Increases joint strength, and, as with most rebounding exercise, improves bone density.

- ° Beneficial even when used in short intervals, especially useful for both warm-up and cool-down exercises.

- ° There is something enjoyable in performing an exercise that can be improved by using music to assist your rhythm.

- ° It is cheap! You need only an inexpensive rope, portable too – take it on holiday with you.

- ° You do not need to master "flash" moves and manoeuvres to derive a good workout. Basic steps will get the job done.

Usual reasons put forward for *not* skipping:

- ° I'm a bit on the heavy/clumsy side.

- ° I have poor co-ordination.

- ° I'll look stupid.

I can appreciate these objections and have come across them frequently, but I've found that invariably that most objectors are often astonished by just how easily and rapidly they become adept at skipping.

Learning a new skill is always rewarding, and learning something as simple as skipping is extremely satisfying, especially if you started out with some measure of doubt. I have taught hundreds of people to skip; some take under a minute, some have taken a lot longer, but they all have one thing in common – they have all mastered it to a degree. To this date I have never had a failure, and while very few of them will ever be mistaken for Floyd Mayweather, they can all skip well enough to get a decent workout from it. Learning to skip proficiently fills you with a sense of achievement – and while it's hardly up there with getting a pilot's licence or learning the trapeze, it is nevertheless a pleasing accomplishment.

Before you start there are three major considerations:

- ° Length, material and quality of your rope.

- ° Surface you will skip on.

- ° Footwear.

ROPES

(Whether rope, leather, plastic, steel or any other material, all are referred to as 'ropes'.)

When you first start skipping, a light leather or PVC rope will suffice. You may later decide to try out heavier ropes or those composed of wire, plastic tubing or beads; these ropes can make increased demands on you, so I'd advise you kick off with the basic variety.

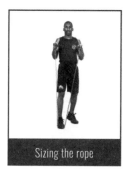

Sizing the rope

Whichever rope you settle on it is vital to have it properly sized.

Ideally a beginner should have a rope they can stand on with the leading foot, where the handles reach the armpits. Extremely tall people may need to get a "made to measure" bespoke version, but given the enormous growth of popularity in skipping (once the sole premise of schoolgirls and boxers, but now widespread in sport) longer ropes can be found online, if not in sports stores. Martial arts stores are often a good source. Shorter people have no such problems; they just need to shorten the rope. Measure the rope by standing on it (as shown), select the right length and simply chop off the excess with scissors or a craft knife and re-secure in the handle by applying a cable tie (available at any D.I.Y store at minimal cost). Err on the longer side at first. You can always cut a little more off – you can't put it back on! Alternatively, knot the end tightly before reinsertion if your rope has wide hollow handles.

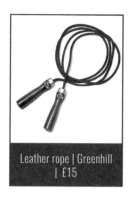

Leather rope | Greenhill | £15

LEATHER ROPES

The original style of rope and still extremely popular, they traditionally have a user-friendly wooden handle and have either a swivel or ball-bearing action for smooth turning.

PVC SPEED ROPES

Intended as the name implies to improve all-round speed. These are generally cheaper to buy than leather ropes.

When trying a speed rope for the first time it would be advisable, in my opinion, to wear track bottoms to minimise whiplash on the legs or hindquarters until you become accustomed to the rope.

"HEAVY HANDS" ROPES

These are designed, or at least intended, to intensify your workout, particularly to the upper body. I would not recommend this type to beginners, but experienced skippers can achieve improved arm strength over a period of time. I would suggest working for short sessions and then build up – or judge by how much your arm aches the first few times!

There are two main versions:

○ Solid metal handles.

○ Hollow handles with removable / adjustable weights.

LONG HANDLED ROPES

Ropes with a long handle make crossovers and other intricate manoeuvres easier to perform; as with many ropes, unsuited to beginners.

CABLE ROPES

These are formed by light, thin strands of metal and can turn incredibly fast for a demanding anaerobic workout. Track bottoms are highly advisable when they are first attempted. This version carries a serious 'lash' for the unwary, which could almost traumatise some users enough to put them off permanently. *Not* for beginners!

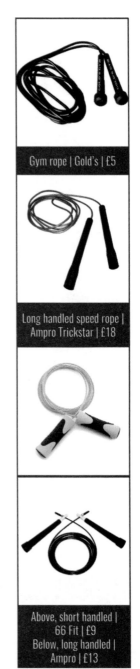

Gym rope | Gold's | £5

Long handled speed rope | Ampro Trickstar | £18

Above, short handled | 66 Fit | £9
Below, long handled | Ampro | £13

THAI ROPES

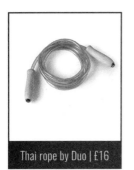

Thai rope by Duo | £16

So-called (unsurprisingly) because they were popularised by Thai boxers, these consist of a "rope" composed of clear, thick plastic tubing. The user soon starts to feel the effects on the arms and shoulders – hard work, but nonetheless rewarding. Start with short sessions and build up. Not for 'learners'.

BEADED ROPE

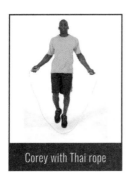

Corey with Thai rope

Composed of cord covered in plastic beads, these are slower to turn but heavy enough to provide a good workout. I found these were well suited to beginners as the slowness gave them control and confidence.

SURFACE

Do not skip on stone, concrete, or other very hard surfaces. The very least you are likely to suffer are blisters on your feet and sore calf muscles. The ideal surface is a sprung wooden floor, or a rubberised gym matted floor. Skipping indoors on carpet is unlikely to prove harmful, but a laminate floor is perfect.

FOOTWEAR

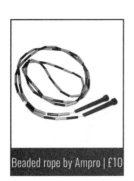

Beaded rope by Ampro | £10

Running, baseball or tennis shoes, cross-training shoes, boxing or wrestling boots are all fine. Make sure your laces are securely fastened before you start as a trailing lace will enforce a stoppage – the lace will impede the rope. If you feel the desire to skip in bare feet, then a judo mat or carpet is user-friendly, a sprung wooden floor is acceptable (for short sessions) but stay away from rock-hard surfaces to avoid blisters.

OTHER CONSIDERATIONS

° Long hair? Tie it back (or it will drive you crazy).

° Loose-fitting spectacles? Secure them around the back of the head with a spectacle strap or lanyard, to avoid watching them take flight across the room. These gizmos cost £2-3. For new specs you can multiply that by at least a hundred.

° You may want to place your drinks bottle within easy reach to sip between intervals of skipping.

° Skip where you can see the clock (you can't glance at your wristwatch), or have a timer with an alarm within earshot. Get a kitchen timer (about £3) or use the stopwatch facility on your sports watch, mobile phone, iPad or similar.

MAKING A START

Be prepared to be a little patient with yourself at first, it may take a few false starts before you become accomplished. A background in dancing, gymnastics or most sports should prove advantageous, but regardless of your background it should not prove too tricky. Never forget, little girls can always do it, usually because they are relaxed and fearless – so get yourself into that mindset.

START-UP POSITION

Where possible stand opposite a full-length mirror. It is important to keep your head up, keeping it in line with your spine, always. To maintain a functional posture resist looking down at your feet to check on how they are getting on. Regulate your breathing by

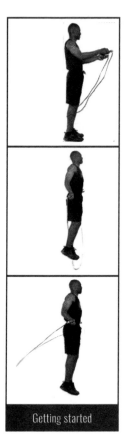

Getting started

inhaling deeply through your nose to 'keep some air in the tank'. Skipping can prove tiring when you first try it out seriously.

Your feet should be slightly less than shoulder width apart, and the rope should rest across your calf muscles

GET A GRIP

Grip the handle firmly but not with a cliff-hanging 'grip of death', and remember – *relax, relax, relax*. Extend your thumb alongside the handle. Note temporary modification to a rope borrowed from a taller person; if you do not want to cut the rope – keep knotting it until you get the right length.

GETTING MOVING

Begin by bouncing lightly on the balls of your feet in a relaxed tempo. Once you have established an easy, almost effortless bouncing rhythm, flip the rope forward over your head, clearing your feet by a few inches with each revolution.

You will, inevitably, hit your feet from time to time, which can be frustrating just as you think you are getting the hang of it. A useful tip when this occurs is *don't stop bouncing.* Carry on without the rope turning to stay in your bouncing rhythm – flip the rope back over your head to the start-up position (on the back of the calves), then start over again. By not stopping and resolutely maintaining your 'bounce' it will serve to improve your rhythm by keeping it constant, help maintain a seamless workout, and hopefully give you added confidence in your ability to keep going. Stopping and starting can be annoying, which is why I stress skipping may take a little patience.

Just like learning to drive or ride a bike, you get better in small increments – and run less chance of injury when you mess up.

MOVING ON

Once you can skip by bouncing up and down on the spot it is time to move on. The bounce is your fall-back 'bread and butter' move, but can be boring due to the constant repetition – develop your own style with some new, uncomplicated moves to give it a little *frisson*.

Modify your style slightly by bringing your elbows a little closer to the body (holding the arms in a wide spread becomes tiring), as this allows the lower arm to do more of the work and is doing so simplify the action, and get better control.

Tip: you may want to stop and give your calf muscles a quick (6-8 seconds) stretch (see "Stretching" for detail) after your first 2-minute session, this area takes the most pounding – which is why it is a good idea to initially wear a running shoe with a cushioned heel.

ALTERNATE STEPPING

Starting out with the two-footed bounce, progress to placing your feet alternately to the front, imagine you are treading out a couple of lighted cigarette butts. Vary this by taking a double beat with each foot.

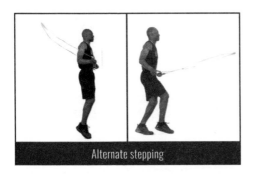
Alternate stepping

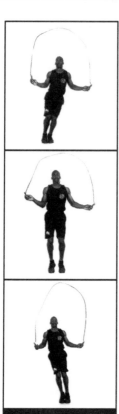

Ski hops

SKI HOPS

Feet together, hop from side to side and backward and forward.

SPLIT STEPS

Feet together, then feet apart – it's as simple as that.

HOP AND KICK

Hop on one foot, then take a small kick forward with the other. The classic-looking 'boxing skip'. Skipping on one leg at a time in a series of hops will give improved leg strength and balance. Try going forward for a short distance in this mode, then back up in similar fashion.

X-LEGGED

Start with the bounce then cross and uncross legs.

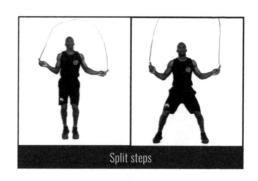

Split steps

LEG RAISE

Work the lower abdominal muscles as you skip by raising the leg to form a right angle (or greater). The effects of this exercise are usually soon to be recognised as it is quite demanding.

CROSSOVERS

Better with a longish rope and the longer the handles the better. Start off by bouncing, then cross your arms in front of you at waist level so that the rope forms a wide loop which you pass under your feet with a downward sweep of your crossed arms. Once the rope has passed under your feet bring your arms back to the start position – *don't change your speed, keep the same tempo.*

It will take a little getting used to before you can impress onlookers with your consummate skills.

RUNNING IN PLACE

This is great for interval training, interspersing periods of jogging in place with flat-out sprinting. If there is adequate space, you can run both forward and backward with varying pace. At my first boxing club this was the only permitted style of skipping, as Ron (our trainer) considered anything else to be 'showing off'. I still feel a pang of guilt doing anything different. However, Ron did teach me an important lesson that I always pass on to novices – "go and watch somebody who is good – and then copy everything they do." That is how *I* learned.

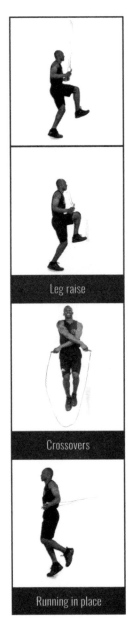

Leg raise

Crossovers

Running in place

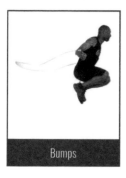

Bumps

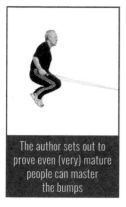

The author sets out to prove even (very) mature people can master the bumps

BUMPS

I've always called this move "the bumps" (there are other names but I think it explains the action). After bouncing, leap high with raised knees (akin to a 'tuck jump') as the rope does a double-spin. See how many you can do continuously until you get that lung-bursting feeling that leaves you in no doubt whatsoever that you are now working anaerobically. This is a great way to finish off a 'running skip' (see above) with an explosive conclusion. Try to beat your previous record every time you do it.

REVERSE SKIPPING

Quite a challenge. Start with the rope resting on your shins and try skipping by turning the rope from front to back, a tricky manoeuvre.

GET RHYTHM

Some upbeat music will always help to give you a sense of rhythm, and alleviate boredom, be it rock, techno, hip-hop or good old rock 'n' roll. Skipping without music is, I feel, almost as bad as dancing without it. Some clubs will not have any music on during training, whereas another will, it is usually the choice of the head trainer – if he is giving advice on sparring he is unlikely to want to shout above loud music. Most gyms play background music that may not be to your liking or tempo. If you don't have to, then don't skip in silence – if nobody else is likely to share your taste get your MP3 player on with the kind of earplugs that don't tumble out.

BE MOBILE

Try not to purely skip in one spot – if you can move around then it is better to do so. Try to move up and down, from side to side, and try going to and fro in a twenty past twelve boxing stance when skipping.

Once you have mastered all the moves listed above try combining them all in your sessions for variety.

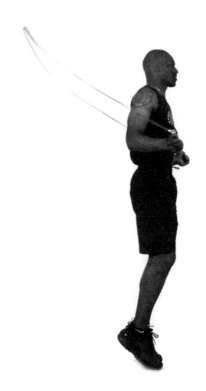

RUNNING

Running is generally referred to as 'roadwork' when applied to boxing training. It benefits both aerobic and anaerobic capacity, according to the intensity applied. It is an established fact that prolonged cardiovascular activities such as running will improve endurance. The run need not be of great length. A functional distance for boxing is around 2-4 miles. If you are a newcomer then once a week will be a good start. For competitive boxing 2-3 runs a week is advisable; professional boxers usually put in 3-5 sessions of roadwork, and many do greater distances. I tend to use the term 'roadwork' to cover other systems of running, as opposed to simply pounding out long continuous runs. Once you have become accustomed to running then it is sensible to move on to something more challenging than simply jogging a few miles – although this is an ideal starting point for novices.

If you are a total newcomer to running, or have not run since you were compelled to in school P.E. sessions, try the following approach.

1. Walk briskly for 3-5 minutes.

2. Jog (slow run) for 3-5 minutes.

3. Stop for a short stretch. Stretch your leg muscles for a few seconds each. All stretching should be done standing: do not lie down for any of the stretches, even if you can, as you are not yet warm enough.

4. Look at your watch and note the time. Run for 7-8 minutes, then turn around and run back to where you started from, tapering off to a very slow pace over the last few hundred yards, slowing gradually to a walk. Walk for 3-5 minutes to cool down, breathing deeply to recover.

5. Once you have come to a stop, stretch again, this time 20-30 seconds. If it is feasible you can do this lying down, preferably on your carpet at home (after checking you do not have mud spattered up your back; I have found this is not well received).

Check how you felt after your initial 15-minute run. If you felt nauseous, exhausted or full of aches and pains, then it will be best to persevere with nothing more than the 15-minute run (or even cut it to 10) until you feel fine after the run. Once you can complete this run comfortably, it is time to move on. Take a couple of days off from running after a session, but not from your other training. You should have recovered completely when the time comes to try another run.

MOVE ON UP

Get your watch on and, using the earlier procedure, progress to doing 20 and then 30 minute runs: the ideal distance. Use the car speedo, sat nav, a local map, or simply the landmarks if you run in a park, to determine how far you have travelled in that time. Try to improve your times. If you want to check on your fitness level, take your pulse at the completion of the run each time.

When you have mastered a steady 30-minute run, try occasionally varying the pace by speeding up for short intervals, alternating with your regular pace.

INTERVAL TRAINING

Interval training consists of periods of extremely hard exercise followed by periods of rest, consisting of flat-out sprints with slow walks in between for recovery. The more unfit you are the longer the rest period you will need. There are many and varied systems of interval training, usually with specific aspects to the discipline they are aimed at, but roadwork for boxing doesn't have to get complicated. For pre-fight training it makes sense to sprint for 2-3 minutes as most training is built around a boxing round duration, with a 1 minute rest, similar to a contest. Ideally you should be completely exhausted at the end of each interval.

Given that information, it may be reasonably concluded that it is extremely hard work, aimed primarily in improving both aerobic and anaerobic capacity. Anaerobic capacity is improved on runs that force you to use up all your oxygen (oxygen debt), and cause a lactic build-up that your cardio system will be compelled to adapt to.

If you are going to try intervals to improve your fitness, which they will, you do not have to be too rigorous when you first start, as the following example shows. Start by running 50 yards/metres – thereafter graduate to 75, 100, 200.

○ After each run, walk back to the start taking deep breaths – this walk is your recovery period.

○ Select a route that has permanent features or markings at both start and finish, e.g. two lamp-posts or trees in a park which are the required distance apart.

○ Warm up first with a jog, long enough to warm your muscles, which will be dependent on the temperature at the time, as well as your body type. Once adequately warm – have a short stretch.

○ Once you are warmed, stretched, and good to go – sprint the required distance as fast as possible. On completion, walk back to your mark; deep inhalations through the nose (more effective than the mouth) will help you recover your breath, hopefully in time for the next sprint.

○ Repeat this procedure for a set number of intervals, possibly 10 to start with.

As you adapt to this discipline, increase the distance and the effort expended.

This is a good way to train with a partner, as you can take turns clocking each other's times to check on your progress. Fiddling about with your own watch to time a sprint is frustrating and usually fruitless.

SPEED

When it comes to speed, we are either the beneficiaries, or prisoners, of our forbears. They have unwittingly determined if we will have fast-twitch muscles (for speed) or slow-twitch muscles (for endurance). Everybody has both types of muscle but some (usually the quicker ones) have more, and often the realisation of this at a young age shapes their athletic prowess. Those with predominately slow-twitch can, fortunately, still improve their speed by training muscle fibres referred to as 'FOG' (fast oxidative glycolic) with interval training.

FARTLEK

This excellent training system is not as popular as it might have been, mostly due to its quaintly vulgar name. It is Swedish for 'speed-play', which would have been such a more suitable title, I am certain, if it wanted to gain serious respectability. It is akin to interval training and can be as hard or easy as you prefer.

It employs varied pace running; mixing up walking, jogging, and sprinting at pre-determined intervals.

Whichever you choose, regarding intervals, it makes a change from other forms of running, and can work on your own or in a group. A popular group running strategy is for all the runners to line up in single file, and at a given signal the back marker must sprint to the front.

Suggested try-out time would be 30 minutes.

HILL RUNNING

Great for endurance training. Made harder than flat running as there is a greater gravitational force opposing you. I take the point some trainers will make that there are no hills in a boxing ring, but if there is a benefit to be derived from an exercise, as there is from hill running, I feel no need to be scrupulously specific.

I realise that not everybody has a user-friendly hill conveniently sited nearby to try hill running, but for those fortunate enough to be adjacent to a hill, or within a short distance of such, it can provide what amounts to a different form of interval training. Start out by running up the hill as fast as possible, followed by a slow descent (downhill running can be unkind to the knee joint), before setting off again. Pump your arms vigorously to assist your effort, increasing your arm speed will assist in increasing your leg speed. Try not to bend your back but maintain a straight spine.

If you want to try this 'Rocky' fashion, by pounding up a steep flight of stone steps, ensure the size and spacing of the steps is conducive to safe foot placement – tumbling down a grassy hill is generally a minor setback; plummeting down a flight of stone steps, however, is an entirely different matter.

SURFACES

If you are a total novice look for parks with a firm sandy path, or a route composed of tarmac – keep away from granite pavements. Sandy beaches look inviting, but unless the sand is hard-packed – avoid it. Soft sand tends to pull on the Achilles tendon.

Seasoned runners might get used to granite pavements, or have little alternative in urban settings and learn to adapt to it, but it is best avoided for newcomers.

Astroturf is a surface I believe is also best avoided, since an osteopath informed me that God invented Astroturf to help his profession prosper. It can play havoc with your hamstrings – a football team I was training got more hamstring pulls on this surface than they ever did in matches.

A hypermarket car park on a summer evening, or after dark if it's floodlit, makes a reasonable (if less than stimulating) jogging track. Sometimes you just have to settle for uninspiring surroundings when seeking a suitable surface, which is probably why my usual run is to circle a tarmac-paved industrial estate.

TREADMILLS

Some people only ever run on treadmills, such is their disdain for road running. If you cannot, or simply do not want to run outside, then the treadmill is the next best thing. If there is an extended period of snow and ice then they are a handy substitute, but I always make them my second choice as roadwork is much more natural. Adjusting to a changing terrain is beneficial to motor skills, as opposed to the steady plod on the treadmill. I never wear an MP3 player during outside roadwork (I want to hear the approach of a juggernaut, a mugger, or that common threat to pedestrians – the adult pavement cyclist), but I feel wearing one is a blessing when presented with the restricted view and monotony of the treadmill. (See chapter on 'Alternative Training'.)

CLOTHING

Recent findings by some sports 'experts' declare that barefoot running is best. Perhaps they are right, but I can only assume they were not intending to doing so in my place of birth – Hackney, East London. Like most urban settings the amount of street debris, ordure etc. makes this suggestion ridiculous. Unless you are fortunate enough to open your front door onto a beach or well-maintained parkland, it is a non-starter. I am a great believer in a maxim that some may now consider archaic: 'football boots for football', 'tennis shoes for tennis' and so on, and would add, 'running shoes for running'.

Your shoes need to be comfortable and do not have to require a visit to your bank manager. Buy them from a dedicated running shop if you can, and if not, from anywhere that will let you try them before you buy them.

Old-time fighters are often pictured running in combat boots (Ali and Sugar Ray Robinson among others) as it was believed that it was beneficial. This practice has died out pretty much now as combat boots, unlike running shoes, are inflexible and tend to place a lot of stress on the knees (not to mention giving you blisters from hell). Functional for the military, who will need to be adept at running in them, but unspecific and pointless for boxing training. Run in comfort.

Do not wear nylon, football-type socks or you could end up with blisters. Cotton socks are preferable.

If you are unsure of the weather (which even British weather forecasters often are), dress up rather than down. A hat can be stuffed into a pocket, a long-sleeved top tied around the waist.

Thin waterproofs are a worthwhile investment. They will not only protect you from the wet, but from the wind as well. Again, this need not cost a fortune, as all the budget sports stores sell waterproofs. You can spring for superior textiles such as Gore-Tex, clima-max, dri-fit and many others – but ask yourself, how often am I going to be running in dubious weather? With any luck a cotton t-shirt and comfortable shorts will suffice.

TIMING YOUR RUN

A digital watch, preferably with a stopwatch facility, is all you need to start with. You will not need Tag or Rolex for your timekeeping – Casio and Timex will do equally well. Most "sports" watches (even the budget variety) have a countdown facility and a 'lap counter' to record your running history. A backlight for those running in the hours of darkness would have an obvious benefit.

DON'T RUN DRY

Unless you want to hump a water bottle around with you (I recently saw somebody running with a plastic 1 litre bottle and thought "that can't feel comfortable"), drink some water a short while before your run to stay hydrated. If you find on your fledgling runs your mouth becomes dry, then try what I prefer and carry a few mints in your pocket to refresh you. Do not, however, overdo it, as too many sweets may cause dehydration – so leave the packet at home and just take a few.

RUN SAFELY

While I would not like to run barefoot in urban areas, neither would I like to run well-shod in them after the hours of darkness, if they were badly lit. Women runners in these areas are ill-advised to run alone, which is something of a sad, but unfortunately true, indictment of our society.

Leaving your mobile phone at home is advisable unless you are going off on what could be tricky terrain in the middle of nowhere – never take this hazard on by yourself, as there is safety in numbers if even the remotest likelihood of accidents seems a possibility. A sprained ankle in the middle of nowhere is not the most enjoyable experience and even worse if you are by yourself. For a run around the park a phone is just unnecessary baggage, especially if you get time-wasters bothering you with unwanted calls about reducing your gas and electricity bills.

CHAPTER FOUR

Another hazard to avoid is an unleashed dog. Certain dogs find moving objects an irresistible challenge, e.g. cats, pigeons, squirrels and, unfortunately, runners. I have suffered two dog attacks; one ankle- nipping (Dachshund), and one knock-down (huge Airedale). My advice is to always give them a wide berth, no matter how friendly they seem – and I speak as a dog-lover.

BOXING DRILLS
SPECIFIC BOXING DRILLS

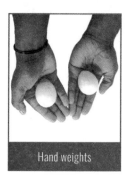

Hand weights

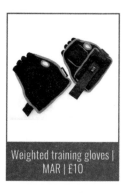

Weighted training gloves |
MAR | £10

There are quite a few drills you can include in your training, which I consider to be not just good fitness exercises but exercises that are functional for boxing.

HEAVY HANDS

Aimed at improving hand-speed and power. It is possible to buy purpose-made gloves for this drill but I feel you are just as well off with the following equipment:

- ○ 2 x 1kg dumbbells

1kg is about right as anything heavier can prove bulky. Expect to pay around £5 a pair. I got these at TK Maxx.

- ○ 2 x smooth stones of virtually the same size, which will fit snugly into the palm of the hand, or, as I have witnessed, a couple of stone or alabaster eggs – perfect fit and perfect weight!

I have seen these eggs online at around £3 a pair.

BOX JUMPS

These improve ankle joint strength as well as push-off power from the rear foot, which is essential in punching and especially with regard to straight punches.

You will need a step box (or similar) which must be sturdy, stable and capable of taking your full weight. The box *must* be placed on a firm surface.

BEGINNER LEVEL

Start by standing alongside the box, then jump sideways and two-footed to land on the box, and then instantly jump to the other side to land two-footed. At first you can gain confidence by taking two bounces both on and off the box. Always land on the balls of the feet.

INTERMEDIATE LEVEL

Once you become self-assured, cut it down to one jump on, one bounce on the box, and one jump off.

ADVANCED LEVEL

Clear the box completely (as shown) with a two-footed jump from side to side. To take it further, try it with two or more boxes, clearing each of them. The intention here is to develop lateral power.

HIGHLY ADVANCED – MIRROR JUMPS

For this killer drill you need 5 boxes and a trainer/motivator to act as a 'mirror'. The motivator faces the jumper and then moves laterally from side to side (he is not jumping anything, just giving you the direction to follow, as you attempt to mirror his movement). Masochists can do this holding hand-weights.

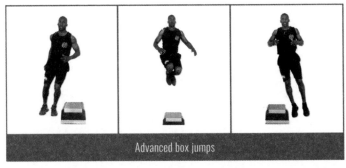

Advanced box jumps

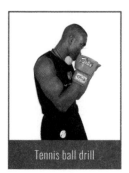

Tennis ball drill

TENNIS BALL DRILL

Try shadow boxing with a tennis ball held in place under the chin in order to adopt the correct head position; very small folk can use a golf or squash ball. Try a session on the punch bag while keeping it in place, then let the ball drop but maintain the same position.

PUNCH BAG THRUST

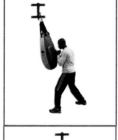

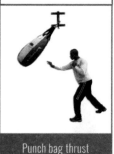

Punch bag thrust

Push a medium to heavy punch bag away with a vigorous shoulder turn, then arrest its return with the same hand in a positive action. Push with the same arm for a set number of repetitions (I would suggest 10 to start with) then switch arms. Make sure no other gym members are within flattening range before launching your 'missile' on your shove/shock routine. This boxing specific drill is listed, as are some of the following, as a "plyometric" drill; most plyometric manuals list exercises for figure-skating, netball, speed-skating and just about every sport imaginable, but I have yet to see one relating to boxing.

DEPTH JUMPS

Intended to 'put a spring in your step' – literally.

Stand on a box 1-2 feet high (a weights bench or two step boxes).

Jump from the box to land softly with bent knees, then explode upwards with arms extended overhead, reaching as high as possible.

After you have mastered this you can add another box to leap over after landing.

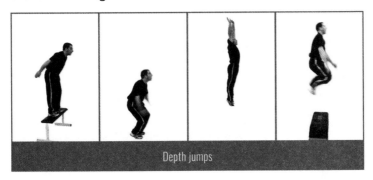

Depth jumps

TUCK JUMPS

Start with your feet shoulder-width apart. Half squat before making a huge leap forward, bringing your knees up to your chest, with your arms holding or touching the knees. Land softly with bent knees.

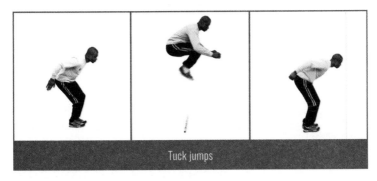

Tuck jumps

BOUNDING & HOPPING

Bounding and hopping improve leg power. If you are unused to this kind of obstacle drill try the action without hurdles before adding them, as both bounding and hopping are still a productive exercise without them.

For boxing footwork, you need to be light and fast on your feet. Exercises such as bounding and hopping can be a great help.

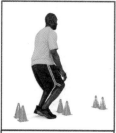

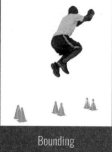

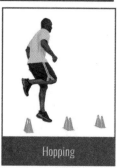

Bounding

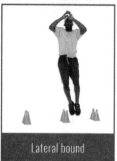

Hopping

Lateral bound

As mentioned in the chapter on technique, punch effectiveness depends on a push-off from the ball of the foot.

BOUNDING

Place some low hurdles (cones or similar) a few feet apart, bound over them to land two-footed – on the balls of the feet. Once you have completed a set of hurdles spin around quickly and come back the other way. This is best done in 'rounds' of 2 or 3 minutes, with a 30 second rest in between.

HOPPING

Taking the same course as above but on one leg, changing legs on the return phase.

LATERAL BOUNDING

Once you have mastered the above, try bounding laterally over the obstacles.

STICK JUMPS

Set 4 sticks on the floor a few feet apart. From a standing start and between two sticks, take off sideways, pushing off with the left foot to land with the right between the adjacent pair of sticks, holding the position for a second before returning. Do 20 repetitions to start with.

This is a good drill to improve lateral movement in boxing.

MEDICINE BALL EXERCISES

The medicine ball is a traditional piece of standard equipment in most boxing gyms. I remember them to be big, furry leather articles incapable of being bounced. There are new and now widely popular balls which are rubberised and come with or without handles.

There are traditional leather medicine balls, old-style – the gym master's favourite missile for miscreants.

The ball without handles is good for bouncing drills, the twin handled ball is beneficial for exercises requiring a firm grip, or one-handed grip.

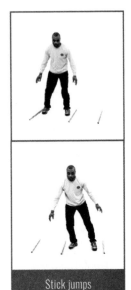

Exercises that require hip rotation are functional for a great many of the movements in boxing. Medicine ball training is excellent for many exercises aimed at improving torso strength and flexibility.

Stick jumps

SIDE TO SIDE BENDS

Hold the medicine ball aloft above your head then bend from side to side to work the oblique muscles, hopefully toning the 'love handle' zone, the oblique muscles.

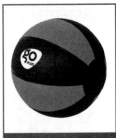

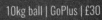
10kg ball | GoPlus | £30

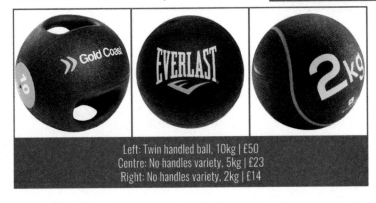
Left: Twin handled ball, 10kg | £50
Centre: No handles variety, 5kg | £23
Right: No handles variety, 2kg | £14

SIDE TO SIDE SEATED MEDICINE BALL BOUNCE AND TWIST.

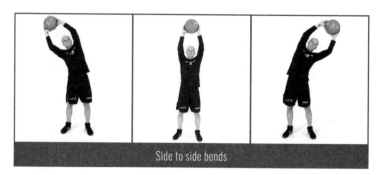

Side to side bends

A challenging abs exercise. Sit on a mat holding a medicine ball. I prefer the twin handled model for this exercise. With knees bent, raise the legs off the floor and bounce the ball from side to side, trying to reach slightly behind you with each bounce.

SEATED SIDE TO SIDE MEDICINE BALL TWISTS.

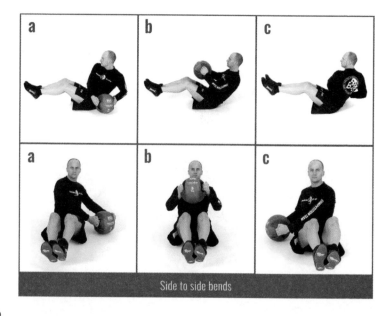

Side to side bends

Similar to the above but without the bounce and with the ball held at arm's length. Sit with legs astride and turn the ball to each side as far as you can.

STANDING SIDE TO SIDE MEDICINE BALL TWISTS.

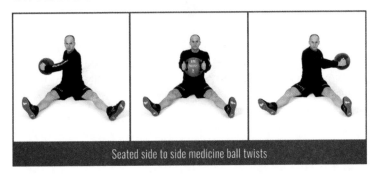

Seated side to side medicine ball twists

Stand with a medicine ball held fully extended, but relaxed, out in front of you. Turn to the side, concentrate on twisting at the hips as if you are about to pass the ball to somebody standing behind you. Come back to the centre each time, pausing 1-2 seconds before the next turn. *Do not twist continuously from side to side.*

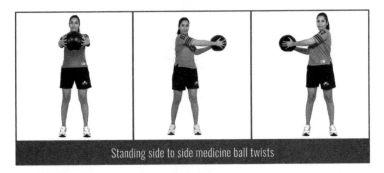

Standing side to side medicine ball twists

PASS-UNDER LUNGES

Combines leg strengthening with co-ordination. Start with the feet shoulder-width apart holding the medicine ball in one hand only. Lunge forward until the lead leg describes a right angle, then pass the ball under the lead leg and into the other hand. Step back and repeat with the other leg.

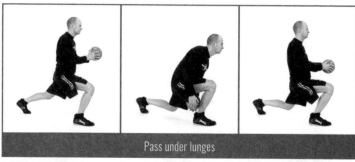
Pass under lunges

MEDICINE BALL LUNGE WALK WITH MEDICINE BALL TWIST

Start with feet shoulder-width apart holding a medicine ball in both hands. Lunge forward, continuing with alternate lunges twisting at the hips on each lunge to extend the ball to the same side as the leading leg. This trunk rotation exercise is excellent for muscles used in throwing hooks as well as strengthening the leg and hip muscles.

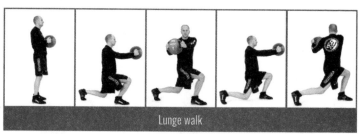
Lunge walk

MEDICINE BALL PULLOVERS

These can be done with or without a ball as you still need to perform a 'double crunch'. Lay on your back with arms fully extended beyond the head holding a medicine ball. Sit forward to bring the medicine ball over your head while simultaneously drawing your knees back towards the body, then 'touch down' between your ankles. Movement should be continuous.

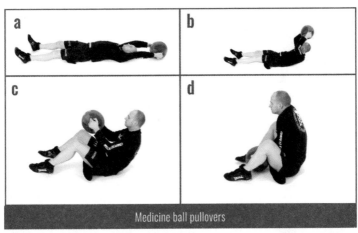

Medicine ball pullovers

MEDICINE BALL PASS-AROUND

Sit on a mat with knees bent and legs raised just off the floor. Pass a light (1-2 kg) medicine ball behind your back and around to the front. Movement should be continuous. Can be done with a set number in one direction then in the other direction, or the trickier manoeuvre, alternating direction i.e. sending it back in the direction it came from.

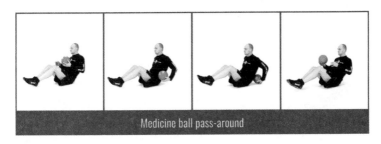

Medicine ball pass-around

SINGLE ARM PRESS-UP

With one arm on medicine ball (or box/step-stool).

Can be performed with several repetitions on each side, or by alternating the arms. For novices, try a few at a time and gradually build up the number of repetitions. Should be performed slowly and in a controlled fashion to avoid wrist injury.

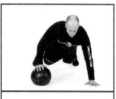

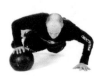

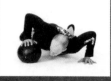

Single arm press-up

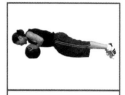

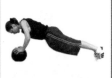

Narrow grip press-up

NARROW GRIP PRESS-UP ON MEDICINE BALL

Use a ball without handles – the squashy type gives better stability. This exercise places greater emphasis on the triceps muscles (back of the arm).

CHOPPING WOOD

Start with feet shoulder-width apart holding the ball in both hands. Drive off with the right foot to swing the ball from low to high and back again. Complete several repetitions on one side then switch to the other side. The foot push-off is excellent training for punching power; the upward torso twist beneficial for the uppercut.

THROWBACK WITH TWIST

This exercise is more demanding than it at first appears and anybody with back problems would be ill-advised to attempt it. You need a rubber medicine ball which is not solid, i.e. capable of being bounced. You will also need a strong flat surface (e.g. the wall of a gym, garage or similar) an unsuited wall could be subjected to structural damage, for this reason I would not encourage anybody to "try this at home".

A 2-3kg ball* is adequate when first attempting this drill.

Stand with your back to the wall with your feet shoulder-width apart. Turn and toss the ball over your shoulder with a powerful rotation of the hips, catch the return and then throw it over the other shoulder. Start out slowly, making lower throws initially if the 'over the shoulder' version turns out to be over-demanding. Novices might prefer to learn the move using a football or basketball.

Once you have mastered the technique fully and become more competent, get into a rhythm as you turn from side to side, and pick up the pace. Larger participants can attempt it with a heavier medicine ball, but no heavier than 5-6 kg, as there is little advantage in using a very heavy ball.

* Illustration, below, shows a 5kg ball being slammed against the wall by a very powerful individual, (my old friend and ex-colleague 'Big Al' Livingstone) – it may take a while to graduate to this level.

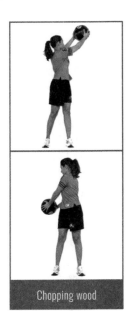

Chopping wood

MEDICINE BALL PARTNER DRILLS

If you have a partner to train with then you can add the following drills to your regime. The ball should not be excessively heavy and should not be the twin-handled variety.

PARTNER PASS-AROUNDS

These can be performed standing or sitting back-to-back with your partner, but I have depicted the standing version for clearer instruction. Stand with feet slightly apart and your arms fully extended, holding the ball in both hands. Pass the ball around to allow your partner to receive it, and then return it in the same fashion. Continue passing the ball around, it is probably more suitable to do for a set time rather than several repetitions.

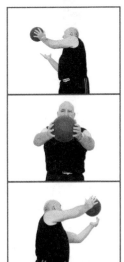

Throwback twist

87

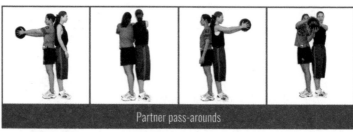

Partner pass-arounds

SHOT PUTTS

Launch the ball from boxing stance single handed to a partner (who *must* be strong enough to catch it) otherwise throw to a mark on the ground. This builds shoulder and arm power. Best suited to throwing with alternate arms to allow for a rest for the non-throwing arm before the next 'launch'.

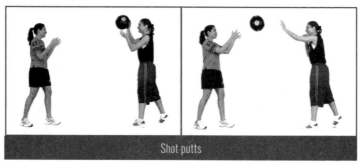

Shot putts

OVERHEAD THROWS

Taking overhead throws with a medicine ball improves your upper body strength; in days of yore footballers would improve their 'throw-in' technique in this fashion, finding it assisted in throwing prodigiously.

Stand with feet shoulder-width apart and release the ball as it comes over your head – your partner *must* be strong enough to catch the ball, otherwise take turns in seeing how far you can throw the ball. When it gets easier start making *small* increments in the distance between you both.

THE POWER WHEEL / ABS WHEEL

This piece of equipment is (realistically) for people who are already well-conditioned, such is its demanding nature. It is designed to improve balance and core stability. The shoulders, chest, back, arms and glutes all get a look-in when working out with the power wheel.

The wheel in basic form (see 'Mini Abs Wheel' below), was first introduced decades ago, and was generally treated with a mixture of hilarity and scorn. It has now made a major renaissance, largely due to the advance of Mixed Martial Arts, many of whose proponents have taken to it with relish.

Abs wheel roll-outs will build a strong core, but must be approached with caution, and it is only proper to point out:

o   You must be warmed up thoroughly.

o   You should have already have attained a good level of fitness.

o   You should use a well-padded surface for knee protection.

o   Only perform a few repetitions in each of your initial sessions (especially if you hope to get out of bed the next day – be warned).

The Lifeline Power Wheel has Velcro-fastening straps and pedals on the side of the wheel to allow you to do press-ups, pikes and the challenging 'crocodile walk', whereby your feet are in the stirrup-like straps as you walk on your hands towing the wheel behind.

The wheel is shown being used in 3 stages:

1. The start position, note the knees are on a padded surface.

2. The halfway rollout. This should be your target when you first start to use the wheel. The distance should then be increased in short increments.

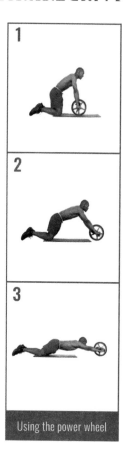

Using the power wheel

3. The full rollout. Note Corey keeps his toes on the floor in order not to put undue stress on the knees.

The training effect is felt very soon after working out, and certainly the next day – it is highly inadvisable to use it on consecutive days unless you are extremely fit.

THE MINI ABS WHEEL

"The Martial Arts Fitness Abs Roller"

There are some variations on the Power Wheel and these small, inexpensive wheels work just fine. With the buzz around core training they have enjoyed an unlikely comeback, and can be found in major gyms – unlike the expensive, albeit vastly superior-build and versatile Power Wheel. A price comparison, in this example from Amazon, illustrate the gulf between the two:

- ○ Lifeline Power Wheel approx. £50

- ○ The Martial Arts Fitness Abs Roller £7.99

The small wheel performs on close to equal terms to the Power Wheel. Working the same muscles when used for rollouts, but lacking the versatility of the bigger wheel for press-ups, pikes etc. It is less of a space-hog, and in my opinion, good value for money.

(All prices quoted as of June 2016.)

TRAINING WITH A PARTNER

It is a boon to have a sympathetic training partner. Together you can work progressively to improve all aspects of technique and fitness. As you become more proficient you will share your ideas and help each other develop. You should both be capable of receiving constructive criticism from your partner, such as "keep your hands up", "keep your chin down," and be grateful for the advice. You can work a system of "one on', one off," whereby you take turns at training drills, with one working hard, one recovering briefly, but exhorting the partner to work even harder.

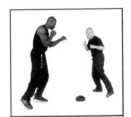

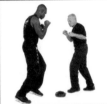

Do not, however, fall into the trap of becoming totally dependent on your partner; have a back-up plan. There will be times, inevitably, when he or she will get stuck at work or in traffic, or on transport, which you should not take as an omen to duck that particularly tough training session. In this scenario work alone to the best of your ability (see 'Solo boxing training workout' chapter).

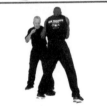

THE DRILLS

Here are some of the partner drills I have used, but be imaginative and develop some of your own. Change them regularly to prevent them becoming stale or boring.

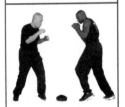

CIRCLING THE PAD

Place a focus pad on the floor and start out

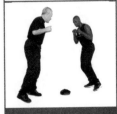

Circling the pad

91

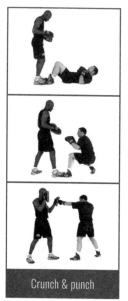

Crunch & punch

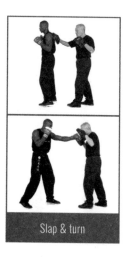

Slap & turn

by facing each other a few feet apart. Move around the pad in a shadow boxing fashion, forcing your partner to retreat in a circular direction. Switch direction frequently and take turns at being the instigator of the movement.

This drill will stop you being a one-directional boxer. Moving around by always going only to the left or to the right, instead of both directions, makes you predictable, and easier to hit.

CRUNCH & PUNCH

The hitter, in bag mitts, starts out by lying in a pre-crunch position, with the pad-holding treading lightly on his toes. After a predetermined number of abs crunches, the hitter leaps to his feet and throws a rapid volley of punches. Start out by doing 10 of each (10 crunches followed by 10 punches) for 3 sets before switching roles. It is harder than it sounds and should be performed in a rapid, anaerobic manner. As you get fitter increase both the repetitions and the sets.

SLAP & TURN

The hitter faces away from the pad-holder, who surprises him/her with a slap on the back. At this signal the hitter spins around and responds to whatever angle the proffered pads are offering, as to whether to jab, cross or whatever punch works the best. This is an all-action, rapid-fire drill, wherein the hitter needs to get into a pattern of hit, turn, hit, turn, with no respite. This should be done in a set number of 2-3 minute rounds, before switching roles.

HIDE THE PADS

The pad-holder moves around with the pads concealed behind him before suddenly producing them, requiring an instant response from his partner.

HIT & RUN

The striker throws a combination of punches in rapid succession, in response to the pad-holder's instruction. The object is for the striker, once the combination is complete, to take evasive action to avoid receiving a (hopefully) light cuff with a pad.

PUNCHING CURL-UPS

One partner lies on his/her back with knees slightly bent. The other partner holds the pads over him/her to start hitting them from a prone position, then gradually withdraws the pads to force the striker to slowly rise in a steady continuous action to make solid contact. Once in a full sitting position the procedure is then reversed, forcing the striker to subside slowly to the floor, still hitting continuously. Predetermine the length of the round and gradually build up intensity and output.

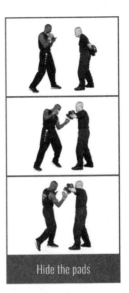

Hide the pads

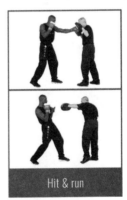

Hit & run

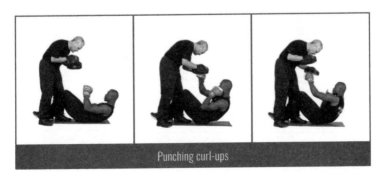

Punching curl-ups

93

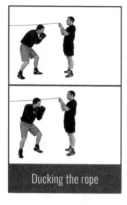

Ducking the rope

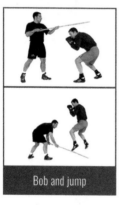

Bob and jump

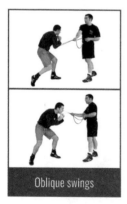

Oblique swings

DUCKING THE ROPE

A length of rope is attached to any convenient fixture (a water pipe was implemented in the example illustrated), at about neck height. One partner lifts and lowers the rope as the other bobs and weaves from side to side, complying with the variance in height. The holder instructs on when to advance and when to retreat. If no partner is available – simply attach the rope at both ends and bob and weave to and fro along its length.

BOB AND JUMP

One partner holds a broomstick (or any slim length of timber), a long bamboo cane from a garden centre is ideal, out in front of him and sweeps it slowly from side to side, both high and low.

The other partner must bob under the high sweeps, and jump over the low ones. Perform slowly and methodically to start with, but progress to sweeping the stick unpredictably to sharpen the reflexes.

OBLIQUE SWINGS

One partner swings a rope (a skipping rope is fine) from side to side going from high to low and low to high, forming a large 'X' shape in the air. The partner avoids contact with the rope by 'angling' in and out of the sweeps. Improves hip rotation for bob and weave technique.

JAB OVER ARM DRILL

This drill is to reinforce sound technique when delivering a jab. The holder offers one pad to be hit, and uses the other pad to form a right angle just below it. To punch cleanly and retract the arm correctly the punch must travel along the correct plane both forward and backward. This drill aims to correct one of the most common defensive failings in boxing, which is dropping the lead hand after landing, or while attempting to land a jab, and thus becoming vulnerable to a right cross.

GLOVE UNDER ARM DRILL

While jabbing with the left hand the hitter must retain a glove under the right arm. This reinforces the importance of keeping the elbow of the defending arm (when jabbing) tucked tightly against the ribs to protect against blows to this area. The lead hand can progress to hooks and uppercuts, but the glove must be retained (on penalty of press-ups or similar penalty, or payment of post training drinks).

LONG & SHORT / SHORT & LONG

The holder extends one pad towards the hitter, the other held in front of his shoulder. The drill is to jab the foremost pad, then by adjusting the footwork, progress swiftly to jab the rear pad. The drill is then changed, the hitter starting with the rear pad then backing up rapidly, always using good footwork technique, to jab the front pad. This is a good drill to perfect the common technique of "stick and move", or the popular colloquial term – "hit and hop it".

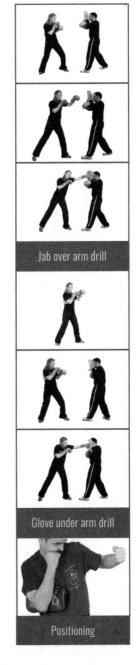

Jab over arm drill

Glove under arm drill

Positioning

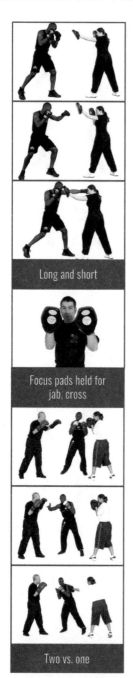

Long and short

Focus pads held for jab, cross

Two vs. one

PUNCHING ENDURANCE DRILL

The holder offers pads purely for jab and cross, as shown.

The drill is simply to complete 3-6 rounds of one minute's duration consisting of continual punching jab and cross, whereby:

- ° Round 1 | Easy

- ° Round 2 | Faster & harder hitting

- ° Round 3 | Fast and hard (4, 5, 6 as 3)

TWO VS. ONE

This is a 'light' drill, mainly for safety reasons, and is best conducted at half pace. It helps with spatial awareness, the importance of footwork speed and sharpens defensive and evasive capabilities. Try a one minute round to start with, then progress to two or even three. I found most people enjoyed this drill as it was usually conducted in a semi-serious manner.

"SHUTTLE" PUNCHING

The hitter throws 10 punches then sets off on a fast sprinting shuttle run for approximately 5 yards (space permitting), then returns to repeat the sequence continuously. Decide beforehand how many, and what variety of punches should be thrown (usually 10, which the holder counts out – loudly), and how long the drill is to last, usually 2-3 minute rounds.

ADVANCED PARTNER DRILLS

This is where you need, ideally, to don your sparring gloves. The big gloves are not only worn to protect your partner's head and body, but to protect your hands, which have a collection of small brittle bones. The defence work on the pad section gives you a basic idea how to defend yourself, but until you start to put the big gloves on and face somebody who is trying to hit you, only then do you realise what a step-up this is. The moves below are a precursor to full sparring, and give you an idea how to build a defence, which is crucial for newcomers to sparring.

DEFENCE DRILLS

(Left-handers to reverse instructions.)

Start out in the basic stance, chin down and eyes up always – and *relax, relax, relax – tension is a hindrance.*

AGAINST THE JAB

Block the incoming jab with your rear hand, held alongside your jaw, 'fielding' it with a semi-clenched glove. Don't slap it away, but instead steer it away from your face. Wait until the jab has passed your own lead hand before blocking, going out with your rear hand to meet the anticipated blow can leave a large gap, rendering you open to a hook-off-the-jab shot.

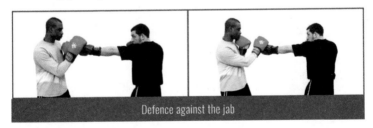

Defence against the jab

AGAINST THE CROSS/ STRAIGHT RIGHT

Steer the incoming punch away with your leading hand, keeping your right hand alongside your face. Note how Wayne, who is throwing the right cross, has retracted his left hand to cover his face (overleaf).

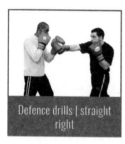

Defence drills | straight right

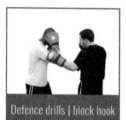

Defence drills | block hook

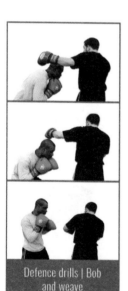

Defence drills | Bob and weave

AGAINST THE HOOK

1. Block with raised arm; as the hook comes towards you raise your arm to provide a solid barrier, while turning away to lessen the impact.

2. Bob and weave; slightly more technical, and best attempted in drills than in your early excursions into sparring. As the hook comes in, 'bob' down by bending the knees and 'weave' (slide under) the punch to allow it to sail over your head, coming up in a position of readiness for a counter-punch. In the example shown, Owen sways from left to right under Wayne's hook and comes up in a perfect position to throw his own hook or cross. This manoeuvre is futile against a much shorter opponent, but it is a great move for a short person engaging somebody who is considerably taller.

3. Sway-back; as the hook swings towards you, simply sway back from the hips to allow it to fall short, sway back into the space you have just vacated to be in a position to counter-punch.

SLOW-MO SPARRING

Just as the title implies, throw all your punches in a slow, deliberate fashion, while wearing 14-18 oz. sparring gloves and mouth guards (gum shields). Agree with your partner beforehand on the 'level of intensity'.

Headguards are a matter of personal choice, but I tend to discourage beginners from wearing them as I feel they give a false sense of security and can lead to a cavalier attitude to head shots, which must always be taken seriously. Some headguards have a poor design and can hinder vision when the head is turned quickly. They should start to be worn when training for competitions in which they are mandatory.

The slow movement can gradually be built up in speed when both of you feel confident enough to do so.

"BACKS TO THE WALL" DEFENCE

Stand with your back to the wall, while your partner throws slow motion punches to your head and body, in a (hopefully) friendly fashion, not unlike the slo-mo sparring (above). Block and evade punches in the manner prescribed above for defence against jabs, straight punches and hooks – without coming away from the wall, you should think of it as 'the ropes'. Do not return fire – no matter how tempting it may be! Start with one minute rounds each and gradually build up to 5-6 rounds of 2-3 minutes each. Well-padded gloves and mouth guards are essential for this drill.

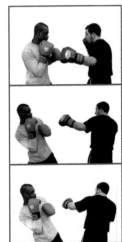

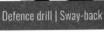

Defence drill | Sway-back

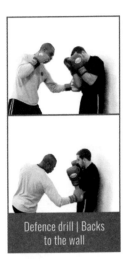

Defence drill | Backs to the wall

THE SOLO BOXING TRAINING WORKOUT

If you are going to train on your own, whether at the gym, or at home, it is best to have a structured plan of action in place. Make a list of the activities you want to do and put them in an order to suit you and your needs. The following is a suggested workout, but many people have used it before going on to tweak it to suit themselves. This workout takes the form of a linear or circular session of circuit training.

EQUIPMENT REQUIRED

- Skipping rope
- Bag mitts
- Exercise mat
- Step-box or sturdy box/crate
- 5-10kg weights (optional)
- Punchbag (any type)

TIPS

- Beginners – halve times/reps where it suits. Take a breather between stations if necessary.
- Advanced – increase times/reps/weights as you see fit. Move swiftly from station to station. Occasionally use a heavy skipping rope.
- Optional equipment extras: power/abs wheel, press-up stands.
- Sip fluids as you go around, and re-stretch if you are feeling tight.

1. SKIP

- ○ 2 minutes

2. SHORT STRETCH

- ○ 8-10 seconds each stretch (all major muscle groups)

3. SHADOW BOX

- ○ 2 minutes

4. PUNCH BAG | ANYONE

- ○ Light and fast punching – 2 minutes

5. SKIP

- ○ 2 minutes

6. ABS CRUNCHES

- ○ 30 reps

7. STEP-UPS

- ○ 30 reps (15 each leg)

8. SKIP

- ○ 1 minute (top speed)

9. PRESS-UPS

- ○ 20-30 reps

10. SHADOW BOX

- ○ 2 minutes (heavy hands)

11. **BOX JUMPS**

- ○ (2 footed jumps on/off box) 1 minute

12. **SQUAT THRUSTS**

- ○ 20 reps

13. **SKIP**

- ○ 2 minutes

14. **HOOKS & UPPERCUTS | PUNCH BAG ONLY**

- ○ 2 minutes

15. **SQUATS**

- ○ 20 reps (hand weights optional)

16. **CRUNCHES**

- ○ 30 reps

17. **PRESS-UPS**

- ○ 20-30 reps

18. **SKIP**

- ○ 2 minutes

19. **HEAVY BAG | IF AVAILABLE**

- ○ Heavy hitting – 2 minutes

20. **LUNGES**

- ○ 20 reps (hand weights optional)

21. SHADOW BOX

- ° 2 minutes (heavy hands)

22. STEP-UPS

- ° (as before)

23. SKIP

- ° 2 minutes

24. TRICEP DIPS

- ° 20-30 reps

25. OBLIQUE TWISTS

- ° 20-30 reps

26. PUNCH BAG

- ° Jab, cross, hook – 2 minutes

27. SKIP | SLOW PACE

- ° (for cool down) – 3-5 minutes

28. LONG STRETCH

- ° 20-30 seconds each muscle group

29. JOINT MOBILISATION

- ° Gentle rotations of neck, shoulders, hips, ankles, wrists
- ° Shake out hands, arms and legs to loosen

WEIGHT TRAINING FOR BOXING FITNESS

Many boxers never include weight training in their regime; Muhammad Ali, Joe Frazier and Roy Jones Jr. are prominent champions who excluded them. Angelo Dundee, who trained Ali, Sugar Ray Leonard and several world champions, disdained them, stating they 'bunched up' a fighter, believing they detracted from elasticity.

Others such as Kelly Pavlik, Frank Bruno and Mike McCallum included them. Evander Holyfield used 'explosive' weight training, and went as far as enlisting a legendary bodybuilding champion, Lee Haney, to instruct him. All this tells us is that some do, some don't – the choice is yours.

I would like to point out that the advice I am giving in this section is intended to help make strength gains to anybody interested in fitness for boxing. It is not aimed at any aspects of bodybuilding; large-scale deforestation must have been required to provide the amount of bodybuilding advice books and magazines. As I'm focusing on boxing fitness I have chosen 'free weights', as opposed to machines, for the following reasons:

○ The movement is more natural, requires utilisation of motor skills, whereas machines have limited planes of movement.

○ Most boxing gyms only provide free weights; it is rare to find Nautilus or similar machinery in a boxing gym.

○ In common with the above, machines require a lot of space; many boxing clubs need all the space they can get for other priorities, i.e. sparring, skipping, shadow boxing and boxing-related exercise.

○ The person who trains at home can get a good workout with an inexpensive set of weights and limited bench equipment. Second-hand weights are as good as new ones.

○ Free weights exercises are self-stabilising, whereas machines provide the stability.

The weights exercises listed are all in free weights, but for the benefit of somebody who wants to use machines (or only has access to machines) I have listed the machine equivalent.

When it comes to weight training for boxing I would always advocate the traditional tried and tested prescription.

LIGHT WEIGHTS | HIGH REPETITIONS

The term 'light weights' would appear a contradiction in terms, but what is light to a 25-stone man cannot be compared with what is light to a 7-stone woman.

It is therefore up to the individual which weights they feel they are comfortable to use for 10-15 reps, for 3 or more sets. If you can only manage a few repetitions of a set weight then it is too heavy, as far as boxing fitness is concerned.

In the photographs describing the movement it can be observed the free weights are comparatively 'light', which I consider is best suited to boxing. Traditionally boxers were told to stay away from weights altogether, as some coaches held a firm belief that they "slowed you down", or "made you muscle-bound", or "made you bulky". Boxers in competition are conscious of their weight, and there is no doubt that lifting heavy weights will, in some cases (not all) make you heavier, not ideal if you are trying to make a certain weight division.

To improve your fitness by adding weights to your regime, I would advise 2 sessions a week (over a 7-day period) – never on consecutive days – unless you are using split routines, which are covered later in the section.

Any regime intended to get you into better shape will almost certainly require some element of resistance training. Simply put, by overloading a muscle you are stimulating it to adapt to the increased load by getting stronger. In the case of most men, due to the presence of the hormone testosterone, the muscle may grow slightly larger, as new muscle fibres are recruited. Men have a much higher level of testosterone than women (it is a

105

steroid androgen formed in the testicles, which may go some way to explain the reason why) which is the simple reason men find it easier than women to grow large muscles. Those seeking bigger muscles should realise that there are factors which govern how much and how big your muscles can grow. Heredity plays a part in this; if your ancestors have bestowed you with larger, fast-contracting fast twitch muscle fibres then muscle growth will be a realistic capability. Do not despair if you are in the slow-twitch group and want to enlarge your muscles – you are just going to have to work that bit harder to get results; genetics may be unfair but never to the extent of being tragic.

The following is a simplistic explanation of why weight training works. If you are presently, or have been recently, lifting weights – skip this bit.

There are many forms of resistance training i.e. the straightforward press/push up, where you simply (simpler for some than others) lift your own body weight from the floor. The weight in this case is whatever you weigh, but by lifting variable loads it becomes possible to gradually increase the load and, in doing so, increase your strength. This can be achieved by using free weights or machine weights. With free weights, you add more plates to a bar or use a larger dumbbell; with machine weights, you set the machine to the next level once the current setting is no longer demanding.

WHY DOES IT WORK?

The simple reason why weight training builds bigger and stronger muscles is, ironically, due to the damage caused by lifting weights. The exercise results in microscopic tears to the muscle fibres, and the repair work the body responds with, which is to enlarge and increase the amount of fibres, as they adapt to the overload. This microscopic tearing is the reason why you will often feel a soreness within the next 48 hours, referred to as Delayed Onset Muscle Soreness (DOMS). The best way to deal with this effect is to always cool down properly, stretch (especially the muscle groups you have been working), and rest from resistance training these muscles for at least 24 hours.

BENEFITS OF WEIGHT TRAINING

○ Builds strength.

○ Improves muscular fitness.

○ Burns off excess fat (by increasing metabolic rate).

○ Increases bone density.

○ Lowers blood pressure.

○ Improves body posture and appearance.

○ Improves sporting fitness (especially when functionalised for specific sports).

○ The "appearance factor" is, I feel, a strong attraction to many who get involved in weight training; it has a knock-on effect, whereby if you start to look better, you start to feel better and renewed self-confidence invariably results.

LEARN THE CORRECT WAY

The best way to get started is to receive instruction from a qualified instructor, so much better than a well-intentioned friend or a book. Books to give you inspiration and advice are plentiful and useful, but you must learn the basics first; just as learning to drive is always better from somebody qualified than from a helpful friend or relative. You ideally need a programme that will be tailored for you, and by telling the instructor your goal he or she must be able to do this – otherwise get a new instructor. Safety is paramount and only an experienced instructor is guaranteed to point out the way to lift weights safely and confidently. See "Safety First" below.

All newcomers to weight training must be aware of the risks involved, injury comes easily when there is misuse or complacency regarding safety, therefore professional tuition is so important – not just for helping you get results, but just as importantly to help you avoid injury.

SAFETY FIRST

Once you have learned to handle weights competently it is worth being aware of the following:

○ If you elect to train at home, keep it as light as possible, especially if you are a novice. Try to train with a partner to assist one another by spotting (tracking the movements of weights, or assisting at the start and finish of moves, and on hand to step in, in case of difficulties).

○ If weights need to be held in place by an Allen Key, spring collar or screw-type collar – check they are tight every time you use them. Falling weight discs and soft footwear are not a happy combination.

○ Only perform recognised exercises as demonstrated by an instructor or listed in respected manuals. Never attempt to improvise or invent moves of your own.

○ Work slowly – this way you will recruit the maximum amount of muscle fibre. You will also have complete control of your equipment, paramount for safety. There are no bone fide exercises that need to be performed hurriedly.

○ Always maintain a straight back. The two most common reasons, in my experience, for people packing-in weight training are:

   ○ Boredom (they have never changed/upgraded their programme).

   ○ They hurt their back through bad technique.

Don't be a hero at the gym. This is mainly a macho thing; the guy who preceded you on the bar just lifted 50k, you don't want to appear wimpy by shifting down to your prescribed 20k, so you make a futile and highly ill-advised attempt at 50k. Don't do this! You may do yourself irreparable harm as you struggle to lift what is obviously an excessive overload. Remember that we all have different needs. Lifting lighter weights should never be regarded in any way as a sign of inadequacy, and it is in fact recommended for most aspects of martial arts and boxing training. If you are unsure of which weight to use then aim low; you can always put more weight on, you can't take it off when you've got the bar stuck at half-way. Just be yourself, ignore other people's weight volumes and techniques, they may have an entirely different agenda – just stick to your own schedule.

Unlike sparring or skipping, don't copy other people – always stick to the way the instructor has shown you. You may espy somebody working out and be tempted to think "that looks good, I'll try it"; this could be disastrous as the other person is likely to be either using an advanced technique, or worse still, incorrect technique.

Be patient. We all progress at different rates. Some people show improvements rapidly; others take months and months. Never despair, it nearly always works if you just give it time.

FREE WEIGHTS

I advocate working in the following order; all exercises have one thing in common – WORK SLOWLY.

The following workout is an all-body routine and you MUST rest the following day to recover and let your muscles adapt. Failure to do so is likely to result in a great deal of soreness.

N.B. Breathing; exhale on the exertion, or use this crude but effective mantra – "blow on the effort".

All weights workouts should be preceded with a warm-up, ideally 5 minutes of cardiovascular exercise, joint mobility, and a short stretch. Stretches should be 6-8 seconds per body part, followed by a cool down, at least a 5-minute cardiovascular exercise, and then a long stretch (20-30 seconds per body part).

This is a very basic "10 Rep Max Workout", which is to say, the first repetition is easy but by the tenth that last repetition should

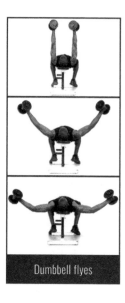

Dumbbell flyes

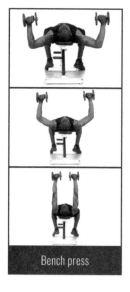

Bench press

be challenging, but never painful. If it hurts – stop, before you cause harm. Always be certain you can lift the weight you intend to work with.

Where applicable I have given (unilateral) single arm working, as opposed to both arms (bilateral), as single arm work appears to be functional for boxing – where punches are thrown one arm at a time.

1. DUMBBELL FLYES | CHEST EXERCISE

Lay on a flat weights bench; if you are improvising at home ensure the bench allows unrestricted shoulder movement (should not be wider than your shoulder blades). Hold the dumbbells directly above your shoulders while maintaining a slight bend in your arms. Lower your arms out to the sides, level with the chest, pause for 1-2 seconds then return to the start point. This exercise targets the pectoral muscles and serves to pre-exhaust the chest prior to the bench press. (See below).

Machine equivalent: 'Pec Deck Flyes'

2. BENCH PRESS | CHEST EXERCISE, SHOULDERS (FRONT), TRICEPS

Laying on the bench as before, begin with the dumbbells out to the side of the chest, or with a barbell held just above the chest. Slowly extend the arms to their full extent, pause 1-2 seconds at the top of the movement, then lower.

A boxing-functional alternative is to lift the weights working the arms alternately.

Machine equivalent: 'Chest Press Station'

3. SINGLE ARM DUMBBELL ROWS | BACK EXERCISE, LATS, SHOULDERS (REAR), BICEPS

Holding the dumbbell at arm's length rest the other hand and knee on the bench (see photo). Slowly raise the arm so the elbow goes as high as possible, then lower to start position. Resist the temptation to "speed up"; some people give the impression they are sawing timber. Avoid this at all costs.

Machine equivalent: Lat Pull Down Station

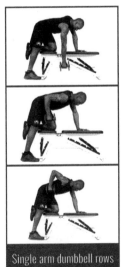

Single arm dumbbell rows

4. UPRIGHT ROWS | UPPER BACK EXERCISE, SHOULDERS (REAR)

Stand with feet shoulder width apart holding the barbell or a pair of dumbbells in front of your thighs. The gap between your hands should be about a hands-width. Raise the weights until they are just below the chin (keep your head back to prevent loosening several teeth). Ensure the elbows are raised higher than the shoulders. Pause at the top of the movement for 1-2 seconds then lower to start position.

Machine Equivalent: Upright Rows on Cable station using straight bar attachment.

5. FRONT RAISE | SHOULDER EXERCISE (FRONT)

Stand with feet shoulder-width apart with dumbbells resting on each thigh, using an overhand grip. Slowly lift the dumbbells one at a time to shoulder level. Do not raise the second dumbbell until the first dumbbell has returned to the start position. This can also be performed by substituting a barbell and lifting it in the same fashion.

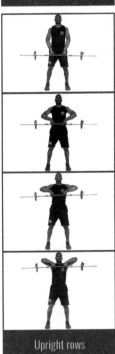

Upright rows

111

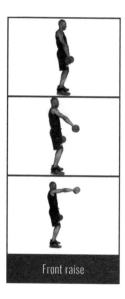

Front raise

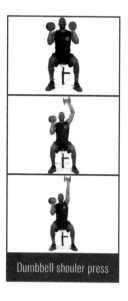

Dumbbell shouler press

Machine Equivalent: not exactly performed the same way, but using the cable station on a low pulley setting allows the same movement, but only by performing alternate sets with each arm, as opposed to the above which uses alternate arms.

6. DUMBBELL SHOULDER PRESS | SHOULDER EXERCISE (MIDDLE, FRONT)

Can be performed standing or seated. I prefer the seated version, as I feel it makes it become more concentrated. Hold the dumbbells just above the shoulders then extend each arm alternately to the full extent of the arm, rotating the wrist just prior to the completion of the movement so that the hand faces inward; pause 1-2 seconds, then lower to start position. Alternative versions are to raise both arms simultaneously or use a barbell.

Machine Equivalent: Shoulder Press Station

7. SEATED BENT-OVER LATERAL RAISE | SHOULDER EXERCISE (ALL)

While seated, bend forward but maintain a straight back. Hold the dumbbells alongside the ankles, with a slight bend in the arms. Slowly raise the arms out to the side, pause 1-2 seconds, then lower to start position. This exercise can also be performed standing in a bent-over position.

Machine Equivalent: Low Pulley Bent-Over Lateral Raises.

8. BARBELL/DUMBBELL SQUATS | QUADS & GLUTEALS EXERCISE

Stand with feet shoulder-width apart with a dumbbell in each hand, held in an overhand grip or with a barbell across the broad part of the rear shoulders, as shown. Look ahead, to ensure a flat back, as you bend the knees until the upper leg is parallel to the floor. Pause 1-2 seconds then return to start position.

Machine Equivalent: Leg Press Machine or Squats using 'Smith Machine'.

9. DEADLIFT | EVERYTHING EXERCISE (LEG & SPINAL MUSCLES ESPECIALLY)

Correct technique is essential when performing a deadlift. The exercise described here differs from the alternative, the 'Stiff-Legged Deadlift', which is an advanced lift only for those with a very strong back.

Stand in front of a barbell in such a way that when looking down you can just see the very front tip of your shoes. Maintain a straight back by looking ahead (never down), then bend the knees and grip the bar with an overhand grip. Slowly lift the bar until it is in front of your thighs – do not bend the arms, but keep them straight. Ensure the shoulders are drawn back powerfully at the top of the list. Pause 2 seconds then lower to within an inch from the floor and continue in this fashion. If this is too demanding, or you are moving on to heavier weights, you can rest the weight back on the floor between lifts. It is possible to perform the deadlift by using two dumbbells but I feel

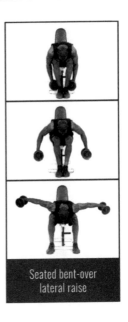

Seated bent-over lateral raise

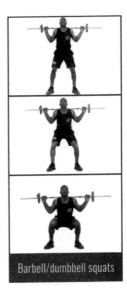

Barbell/dumbbell squats

113

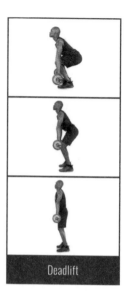

Deadlift

using a bar is more effective.

Machine Equivalent: Deadlift on the 'Smith Machine'.

10. DUMBBELL BICEP CURLS | BICEP EXERCISE

There are many variations on the same theme, but I have gone for the basic dumbbell curl with both weights raised simultaneously; this is to demonstrate the arm action, but I advocate lifting the dumbbells alternately.

Sit (or stand) with the dumbbells hanging down by your sides then slowly raise them by bending the elbow towards the shoulder. Pause 1-2 seconds then lower to start position.

Machine Equivalent: bicep curls on Curl Station or on cable station (ideally using E-Z curl bar, which rotates and is shaped especially for this exercise).

11. SINGLE ARM SEATED TRICEP EXTENSIONS | TRICEP EXERCISE

Sit (or stand) holding a dumbbell (a light one if this is the first time you have attempted this exercise), at arm's length above your head. Reach across with the other arm and hold the bicep, this should stabilise the lower arm during the movement to follow. Slowly lower the arm at the elbow out and behind you, finishing behind your neck. My top tip here, which is less ridiculous than it may seem, is to avoid bringing the weight down on top of your head – I've seen it done. Pause 1-2 seconds then return the arm to the starting position.

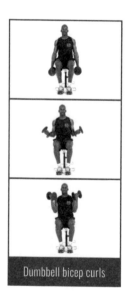

Dumbbell bicep curls

This can also be performed by holding a dumbbell in both hands.

Machine Equivalent: Triceps Press-Down Station or Pushdowns on the cable station, using straight bar or rope attachment.

12. BARBELL CLEAN & PRESS | SHOULDER EXERCISE

Combine working the upper and lower body in the same exercise with this classic lift. Start by standing behind the barbell, ideally an Olympic barbell, with feet shoulder-width apart. Just the tips of your toes should be visible from above and your shins close to the bar. Bend the knees to start the lift, hands taking an overhand grip a little wider than shoulder-width, while keeping your head up to maintain a safe back position.

Performing this exercise in front of a full-length mirror is very helpful. Lift the bar in one fluid movement to shoulder height, flipping the palms of the hands over backwards to support the bar, which should rest on the upper chest prior to the upward overhead press, in which the arms should be fully extended. Reverse the procedure to lower the bar back to the chest, then flipping the hands forwards, lower the bar to the floor. Start with an unloaded bar as a rehearsal; in the first few sessions attempt a limited number of repetitions, adding more as you grow accustomed to the exercise.

Machine equivalent: Smith Machine.

THE OLYMPIC BAR

Using the Olympic bar without any plates

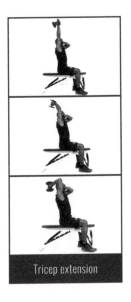
Tricep extension

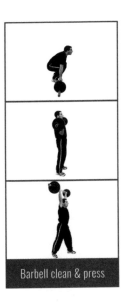
Barbell clean & press

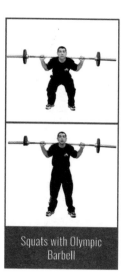

Squats with Olympic Barbell

for this exercise is still beneficial, and will allow for more repetitions. The bar is similarly useful for squats and deadlifts (see above) whether loaded or unloaded when it weighs 20-25kg.

Standard Olympic bars are just over 7 feet / 2.2 metres and weigh 20kg.

Spinlock collars weight roughly 2.5kg each.

SPLIT ROUTINES

I would envisage these to be 'overkill' where boxing fitness was concerned, but *should you get the weight training bug (many do) and decide you want to train a little harder* and more often, you may have to split your training up.

Performing an all-body workout is the ideal starting procedure, but after a while you may feel the need to intensify your training and you cannot as your all-body routine always needs a day off for recovery. The same routine should never be performed on consecutive days. The answer is to split your training into different routines whereby some of your muscles get a rest, while others are working. You need to work out which muscles to train on which days, so no muscles get worked on consecutive days. This may, however, suit people who can only get to the gym on two consecutive days.

There is a substantial amount of reading matter on this subject, both in books and the great many weight training and bodybuilding magazines available. Always try to get hold of up-to-date literature as some of the older books and periodicals give well-intentioned advice which has been outdated, and in some cases as far as instructors go, outmoded or worse still – dangerous. (See "Useful Literature").

Below is a basic two-day split training routine.

DAY 1 AND 3

- ○ Dumbbell Flyes

- ○ Bench Press

- ○ Lat Pull Downs/ Single Arm Rows

- ○ Bicep Curl

- ○ Triceps Pressdowns / Dumbbell Triceps Extensions

- ○ Abdominals (crunches)

DAY 2 AND 4

- ○ Squats

- ○ Deadlifts

- ○ Shoulder press

- ○ Front raise

- ○ Bent-over lateral raises

- ○ Upright rows

- ○ Abdominals (reverse curls)

KETTLEBELLS

Although I knew they were favoured by Russia's special forces, kettlebells were something I first viewed with some scepticism. I have now come to believe they can play an important role in strength and conditioning training. The kettlebell is classified **117** as a free weight, and like the dumbbell is ideal for functional unilateral work.

I would advise anybody who considers some serious training with them to get tuition from a qualified instructor on safe and proper technique – you would not want one of these articles landing on your foot.

I particularly like them for squats and deadlifts, as ably demonstrated below by renowned kettlebell guru, Steve Wright.

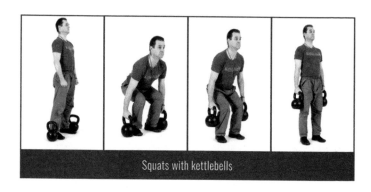

Squats with kettlebells

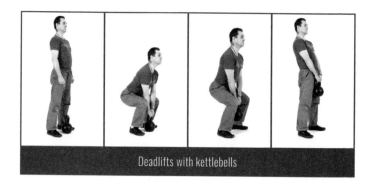

Deadlifts with kettlebells

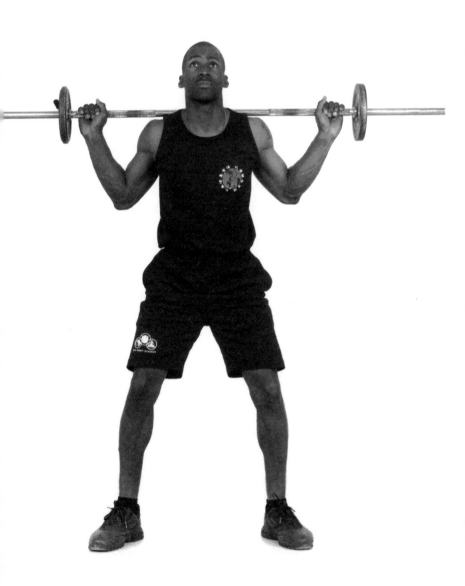

CALISTHENICS & BODYWEIGHT EXERCISES

The term Calisthenics (sometimes spelled *callisthenics*) is a term which tends to be used more in the USA than in the UK. It comes from the Greek words 'kallos' (beauty) and 'sthenos' (strength). For now, we are going to skip the beauty part (too late in the day for many of us) and home in on the strength element.

Bodyweight exercises are perfect for beginners, and should not be sneered at by experienced practitioners as they are of great value.

Many successful and highly trained professional boxers solely depend on bodyweight exercises; Muhammad Ali, Jack Dempsey, Joe Louis and Sugar Ray Robinson (probably the finest of them all) excelled without ever considering weight training.

I would advocate bodyweight exercises for the following reasons:

○   They are versatile – you can train all body parts.

○   Bodyweight training is free – no need to go to a gym or club, as they can all be done at home.

○   It teaches good form and balance for exercises such as squats and lunges, prior to the addition of weights to perform these exercises.

○   Adding a minimal amount of equipment, a box/step and stands for press-ups, adds to the range and scope of exercise.

In the following exercises I have included some with a medicine ball or a bench, as most gyms/clubs make them available. For home training a sturdy box, step-stool and a football or basketball can be substituted if a medicine ball is not available.

THE EXERCISES

1. PRESS-UPS

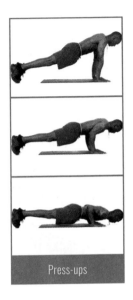

Push-ups in the USA, but just as effective (if demanding) no matter what term is given to them. They are easy to explain but as all schoolboys remember, hard to perform in a large number of repetitions (especially if under the critical eye of a PE teacher).

The resistance is provided by travelling upward against gravity; merely standing upright in front of a wall performing this exercise would be easy.

Press-ups

Keep the body straight, head in line with the spine, and start with the hands under the shoulders. Slowly lower your body until your nose is practically touching the floor, and then push your body back to the start position, slowly – and without holding your breath; try to breathe normally all through the exercise.

Variations include wide and narrow grips to place emphasis on different areas of the chest, shoulder or triceps, the main muscles involved.

MAKING PRESS-UPS EASIER / HARDER

Easier

If you are unfamiliar with press-ups then an easier introduction is performing 'box' press-ups.

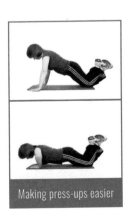

Making press-ups easier

Start with bent knees (as shown), so always use a mat/carpet, as your patella (kneecap), which is not much bigger than a £2 coin,

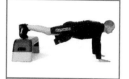

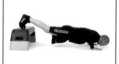

Making press-ups harder

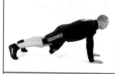

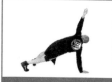

Rotational press-ups

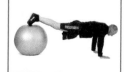

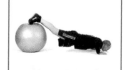

Press-ups with a swiss ball

should be cushioned from a hard surface to prevent soreness or injury.

Harder

By raising your feet, the exercise becomes more difficult, and more productive. If you do not have a box/deck, then use **a step** or stair in your home.

2. ROTATIONAL PRESS-UPS

Rotation plays a large part in boxing; hooking, upper cutting and evasion manoeuvres in particular. Perform a press-up then turn and extend one arm while supporting the body, as depicted. Return to the start, execute another press-up, then rotate in the opposite direction.

Tip 1

Introducing an unstable surface, such as placing either the feet or hands on a Swiss Ball or medicine ball, will involve the back and rear shoulder muscles.

Tip 2

Introducing a pair of 'press-up stands' takes the pressure off the wrist joint and allows for a deeper descent.

3. CURL-UPS, REVERSE CURLS & CRUNCHES

The above exercises target the abdominal muscles, and you'll notice I have excluded the term 'sit-ups'. Although it is still used in some circles as a catch-all phrase for abdominal exercises it should be noted that, if the lower back is lifted off the floor to perform the action during supine abdominal exercise, then the hip flexors do the bulk of the work. Full sit-ups are not particularly good news for the back, and require a good standard of fitness to be performed functionally i.e. to strengthen the hip flexors, and should be performed sparingly. Many 'old school' exercises have been making a comeback lately and there is a school of thought that sees merit in full sit-ups, but I am still not convinced they are beneficial.

I often see curl-ups described as crunches – and vice versa, but if the knees are bent and the lower back stays on the floor, then only the abdominal muscles should be engaged.

I must point out that doing these exercises will *not help you to attain a set of abdominal muscles that resembles a tray of ice-cubes*. What it will do is help, in addition to other 'core' exercises, to give you a powerful midsection – invaluable in boxing. 'Spot reduction' (repeatedly working one area of the body to lose weight) is a non-starter, and your six-pack will only be visible once body fat from all over the body has been reduced. To many people this is regrettably due to dietary reasons more than those concerning exercise.

Tip 1

Do not pull on your head – it will give you a sore, stiff neck and ruin your body-shape when performing these exercises. Instead, rest the fingertips against the temples, or to make it a little easier, fold the arms across the chest.

Tip 2

In these exercises try to contract your abdominal muscles, but breathe naturally – never hold your breath.

CURL-UPS

Lay on your back with knees bent and feet apart, and then slowly curl forward, raising just the shoulder blades off the floor, then return slowly to the start position.

REVERSE CURLS

This exercise targets the lower part of the abdominal muscles. Lie on your back with your hands close to your sides. Your legs

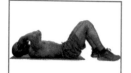

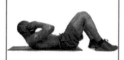

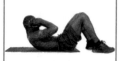

Curl-ups

should be bent at the knee and crossed at the ankles (or simply touching if the former is uncomfortable). From this position, slowly lift your hips off the floor by bringing your legs towards your ribcage. Once your hips have cleared the floor the upward movement is completed. Slowly return to the start position.

CRUNCHES

Crunches involve raising the legs to isolate the abdominal muscles for them to take more of the load than the hip flexors – especially if you maintain the leg position and keep your backside close to the box while lifting the shoulder blades off the floor, not the lower back.

OBLIQUE TWISTS

The oblique muscles are found on either side of the abdomen, and according to their shape and size (occasionally over-size) are often described as 'love handles'. These twists are also referred to as 'twisting sit-ups' (even in the excellent *The Concise Book of Muscles* by Chris Jarmey).

In this exercise, you start out laying on the floor with bent knees and your fingertips lightly touching your temples.

The feet stay on the floor as you slowly raise the trunk, leaving the lower back on the floor, then twist the trunk while lifting the opposite knee to bring them together.

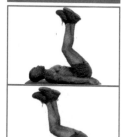

Reverse curls

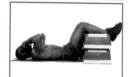

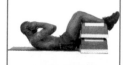

Crunches

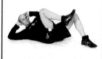

Oblique twists

DOUBLE CRUNCH

Lay on your back on a mat with knees bent and fingers resting lightly at the side of the head. Bring head and shoulders forward and raise the legs simultaneously to meet the elbows. Note (below) that Dave's lower back stays on the floor at every stage.

LOWER ABS 'TUCKS'

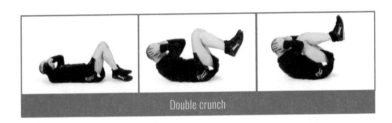

Double crunch

° With a medicine ball

Sit on a mat with a medicine ball held between your knees. Lean

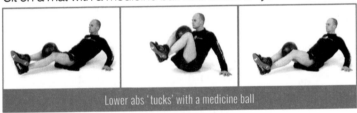

Lower abs 'tucks' with a medicine ball

back 45 degrees, supported by your hands. Raise your legs and draw the ball towards your midriff.

° On the end of a bench/box or similar

Sit on the end of a bench with your legs extended in front of you. Draw your legs back towards your midriff.

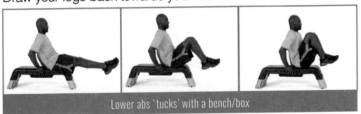

Lower abs 'tucks' with a bench/box

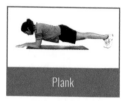

Plank

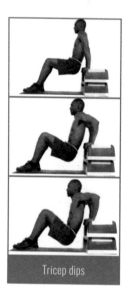

Side plank

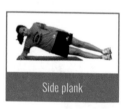

Tricep dips

THE PLANK (BRIDGE)

This is a staple core training exercise which, apart from working just about all the abdominal muscles, gives muscular stability which is invaluable in combat sports such as boxing.

Lie face down on a mat supported by only your elbows and toes. Your arms should be at right angles with your elbows directly below your shoulders. Use a mirror or ask a friend to check that your body is parallel to the floor. Keep your spine neutral and your head in line with your spine. Contract your abdominal muscles, but do not hold your breath; breathe normally. Try to hold the position for as long as possible, starting with 20-30 seconds and building up gradually with each session to 2 minutes.

There are two versions, the front plank and the side plank.

This version targets the oblique muscles, and most folk find it harder than the front plank. Raise yourself up on one elbow, with the arm bent at 90 degrees, your other point of contact with the floor being the side of your lower foot. As with the plank, hold as long as you can.

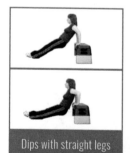

Dips with straight legs

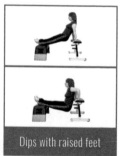

Dips with raised feet

4. TRICEP DIPS

For this exercise you need a sturdy box, step stool, or a stair. Place your hands behind you, with the heel of each hand firmly gripping the edge of the surface. Bend your arms at a right angle and then push up again to the start.

Doing this with straight legs makes it harder, as does propping the feet up.

5. CHINS (CHIN/PULL-UPS)

An exercise more suited to featherweights than heavyweights as far as the number of full repetitions go.

Grip an overhead bar in either an overhand (pronated) or underhand (supinated) grip.

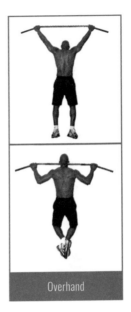

Overhand

In the underhand grip there is assistance from the bicep muscles; this is not the case in the overhand method, where there is little assistance from the arms and the back muscles, lats, trapezius, teres and rhomboids, do most of the work.

6. LUNGES

The lunge, when performed without weights, is particularly beneficial for developing balance and co-ordination, and stretch the hip area if they are performed correctly, i.e. with the upper body erect and the front leg should form a right angle,

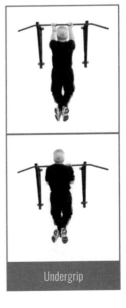

Undergrip

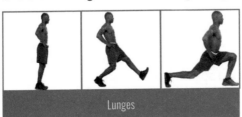

Lunges

127

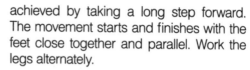

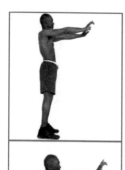

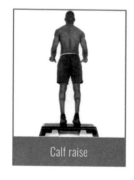

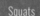
Squats

achieved by taking a long step forward. The movement starts and finishes with the feet close together and parallel. Work the legs alternately.

If you are not confident at first then simply extend your arms to assist balance, akin to a tightrope walker. Keep your head up and maintain good alignment throughout.

7. SQUATS

A great weights-free version of the squat, and a good introduction to anybody considering reforming it with weights.

Aim to squat to a depth whereby your upper leg is parallel to the floor. If this is not achievable when you start, simply bend as deeply as you can and try to gain a little more each time you train. A less than parallel squat is better than no squat at all if you are trying to get fit. Novices can support their heels on a weights disc if it helps.

Extend the hands out to the front to assist with balance. Note in the illustration, above left, how far back Corey's body weight is, and his toes are turned slightly outward for stability.

8. CALF RAISE

Stand on a sturdy box or step in such a way as you can get support from a wall or rail. Only your toes should be in contact with the box. Go up on your toes, then drop your heels slowly until they hang slightly below the box. Strengthens the gastrocnemius and soleus, the large calf muscles.

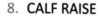
Calf raise

9. STEP-UPS

Utilise a box, step-stool or stair and lead with either foot in order to form a right angle. It is more time and energy efficient to do a set number of repetitions on one leg and then do the same with the other leg – working the legs alternately tends to be a slower procedure. Once you become confident there is no longer a need to look down to check foot placement – try to keep your head up.

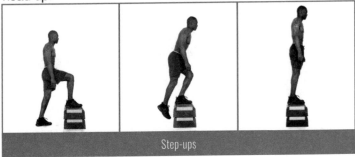

Step-ups

10.BACK EXTENSIONS

Lie face down on a comfortable surface; if it's not comfortable when you begin it's unlikely to improve after 10-15 repetitions. Slowly raise the upper body, as shown below. This exercise strengthens the spinal erectors of the back.

11.SQUAT THRUSTS & BURPEES

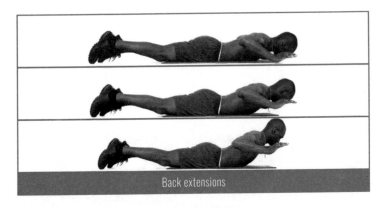

Back extensions

These exercises will take many people back to school PE, both staples in the regime of school exercise. They use just about every muscle area going: the arms, legs, abs in particular.

SQUAT THRUSTS

Squat with your hands in front of you, then, supported by your hands, thrust your legs backward with an explosive action, then return your knees to come between your arms, the start position.

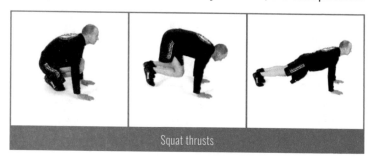

Squat thrusts

BURPEES

A variation of the above that makes it a little harder. Start out by standing up, drop into the squat thrust start position, perform a squat thrust, then jump briskly to your feet before starting all over again. Variations include inserting one or more press-ups before the jump-up, or substituting 'tuck jumps' or 'star jumps' for the basic jump-up. The military love them, as do many martial arts instructors – but if you come to despise them (schoolboys inevitably did) then the blame goes to an American physiologist, Mr Royal H Burpee.

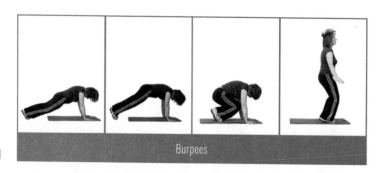

Burpees

12. VAULTS (ON STEPBOX/BENCH)

For this exercise you will need a sturdy box or bench around 18"/35cm high. You can elect to use a higher bench, but it will make it harder to clear.

Stand alongside the bench leaning forward and grasping the bench firmly on each side. With feet together, vault the bench from side to side with a dynamic sideway jump. The emphasis is on the arms and shoulders, but it is pretty much a whole-body exercise.

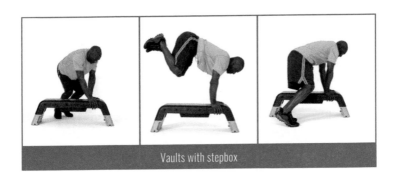

Vaults with stepbox

CORE TRAINING | THE SWISS BALL

Core Training – training the muscles of the torso which provide stability – has become commonplace in most gyms now. Although it was unheard of in this form, most people were doing some kind of core training (e.g. press-ups and crunches) as part of their fitness routine. The introduction of the Swiss Ball gave a new dimension to this kind of training, and although I sneered at it originally, I have come to use it in training with an increased frequency over the years.

Building a powerful core is essential in boxing, as well as making everyday physical tasks, such as lifting and carrying, easier to accomplish.

There is a great deal of equipment currently in use when it comes to core training, some basic, some quite sophisticated. There is a great deal of splendid material devoted purely to core training; this is *not a core training manual and I have attempted to make the exercises boxing-specific.* I have selected the Swiss Ball (and occasionally medicine balls) for this book, for three main reasons:

- It fulfills the needs of boxing fitness pertaining to the core.

- The Swiss Ball is accessible. Most gyms have one.

- The Swiss Ball is affordable for home training. They range in price from around £6 to £30 (I have to say that personally I have found the quality is reflected in the price – I had two cheap balls that punctured easily, but a £24 'Fitness Mad' ball has proved excellent).

This item of equipment goes by various names – the Fitball, Stability Ball, Medi-ball, Physio Ball and the Gym-ball are just some other variations I have heard, but it was first introduced as the Swiss Ball, so I'm sticking with that.

I am informed it was first introduced by Swiss remedial therapists to assist primarily with back problems, and was treated at best with curiosity, and oft-times with derision on its earliest ingress to gymnasiums. It has nevertheless grown in popularity due to the variety of exercises it allows and its effectiveness. You use a numerous amount of muscles merely to stop yourself falling off the thing.

The extra effort required to manage the additional element of instability allows for core improvements both in strength and balance. The idea is that the unstable surface will place additional emphasis on the trunk muscles in order to provide improved spinal balance and stability. It takes a little getting used to at first and I would suggest using it on a soft surface to begin with – just in case. It may not be far to fall if you tumble off, but a cushioned floor is better for both you and the ball's longevity as they can be vulnerable on rough surfaces.

There are many volumes dedicated to Swiss Ball training (see "Useful Literature"), but in this section I have listed some exercises I think suited to boxing fitness.

KNOW YOUR LIMITS

Do not try any complicated exercises until you feel completely confident laying backward on the ball. In many gyms the Swiss Ball has been used as a substitute for the weights bench; this is all well and good, provided the weights are *not heavy – if they are it is far better* and safer to use a bench. I've never seen anyone fall off a bench with weights in their hands, but I've heard cases of this happening on Swiss Balls when excessive weight was used. I have never yet heard of a bench bursting or being punctured. However, rarely, this may happen to a Swiss Ball. It is usually where some imbecile has left a sharp object lying about on the floor. There is no hard evidence to support weight training on the Swiss Ball is superior for muscular improvement – if using heavier weights for muscle gain you are better off on a bench – the ball's prime use should be to improve *stability.*

I also strongly advise against standing on the Swiss Ball. Kneeling on the ball in a safe environment, i.e. on a carpet or a judo mat, is an aid to improving balance, but standing on the ball carries no benefit that is worth the high degree of accident liability.

Make sure your ball is always fully inflated (the cheaper, thinner-skinned models seem to deflate more quickly) and keep it well away from sharp edges of gym equipment, tools or furniture.

GET THE SIZE RIGHT

The following is a general guide used by most Swiss Ball retailers, and I have found it to be reliable:

USER'S HEIGHT		BALL SIZE
ft / in	cm	cm
4'8" – 5'5"	140 – 160cm	55cm
5'6" – 6'0"	165cm – 180cm	65cm
6' +	180cm +	75cm

Most manufacturers state that the maximum load is 300kg, and although I'd advise against putting this to a practical test I do know of a physiotherapist, a 30-stone giant of a man, who uses his as an office chair in relative comfort.

As stated previously there are numerous books and DVDs dedicated to Swiss Ball exercises, but in the following section I have provided a basic workout functional for boxing.

1. WALL SQUAT

Place the ball between a wall and your back and, looking ahead, keep your body straight and bend into a squat position until your thighs are parallel with the floor. Hold for 1-2 seconds and then return to start position. Keep the pressure on the ball by constantly leaning back into it to retain it as it rolls up and down with you.

2. PRESS-UPS

There are two different press-up techniques which can be employed; both are (in my experience) challenging.

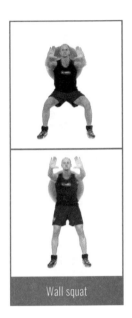

Wall squat

○ Rest your hands firmly on the ball, ensure your body is straight (check in the mirror or ask somebody). Lower your chest down onto the ball, pause 1-2 seconds and return to start position. The slower you work the more control you should have.

○ Place your insteps on the ball and, ensuring your body is straight, lower yourself to the floor, pause 1-2 seconds and then return to the start position. To make it more challenging try to do this with the tips of your toes on the ball.

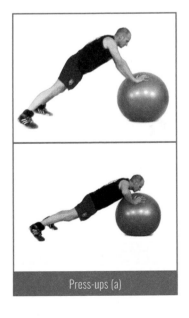

Press-ups (a)

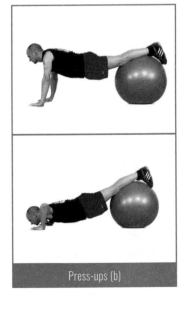

Press-ups (b)

135

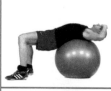

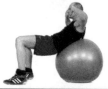

Curls

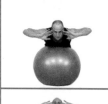

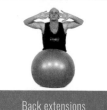

Back extensions

3. CURLS

Begin by sitting on the ball. Slowly walk your feet forward, allowing your lower back to come to a rest on the ball. With just the tips of your fingers touching your head, progress to now curling your body upward, then slowly coming down again. Pause for 1-2 seconds at the top and bottom of the exercise. To make this a little more demanding you can hold a medicine ball.

4. BACK EXTENSIONS

Lie on the ball resting on your mid-section. With your elbows out to the sides (as if giving a double salute) slowly lift your upper body, pause for 1-2 seconds, then lower to the start position.

5. RUSSIAN TWISTS

Lay on your back on the ball in the same start position as curls (no.3). Fully extend your arms above you. If you do not have a medicine ball, football or dumbbell simply place the palms of the hands together. Roll to alternate sides, coming to rest on the shoulder at the completion of the turn.

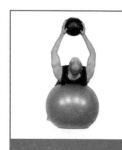

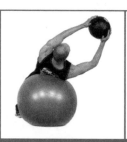

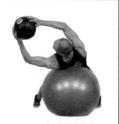

Russian twists

6. JACK-KNIFE

These are also referred to as 'reverse roll-ins'; start as if about to do a press-up with the legs on the ball (see photo). Bend your knees to roll the ball toward you. Pause 1-2 seconds then roll the ball back by extending your legs.

7. LATERAL CURLS

Lay sideways on the ball with the elbows out to the side giving a double salute. If this is difficult at first, try holding onto the ball with the lower arm, instead of bending the elbow. It may also help to start with your feet against the base of a wall. Once you are in position raise your upper body sideways as far as you can, pause1-2 seconds, then return to the start position.

8. PLANK

Rest your hands on the Swiss ball in the same position as you would to perform a press-up. Contract your abdominal muscles but don't hold your breath as you maintain a stable position for as long as you can.

9. KNEELING ON THE BALL

A demanding balance test. Make sure you are next to a wall or a stable surface (I prefer the stack of judo mats). Start with the ball on a judo mat or a large gym mat if this is possible – please do not attempt this where there is a concrete floor! Climb onto the ball with both hands and one leg, then hoist the other leg onto the ball, holding on to the wall for support if you feel unstable. Try to let go of your support as you come up into a kneeling position with your arms

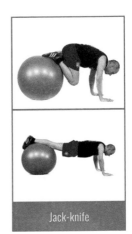

Jack-knife

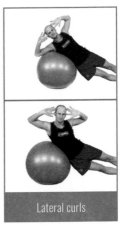

Lateral curls

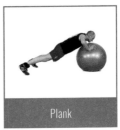

Plank

outstretched for balance, akin to a tightrope walker. Use a timer to see how long you can last, always striving to beat your previous best. As mentioned previously, resist the desire to stand up on the ball. The danger outweighs any benefit.

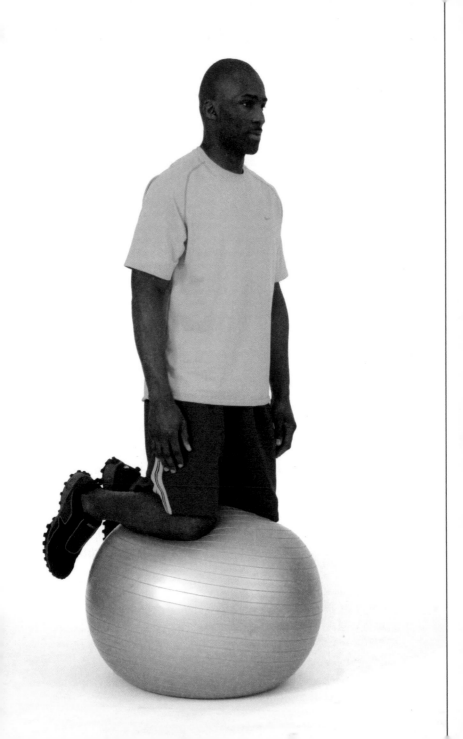

FLEXIBILITY & STRETCHING

Maintaining flexibility, especially as we get older, is important. It can improve your performance regarding physical activity as well as in your day to day tasks. It should also reduce the risk of injury. Post-exercise stretches will speed your recovery from training, in addition to maintaining or even further developing your level of flexibility.

Thus, your training should usually encompass the following phases: the warm-up; the workout; the warm-down; the warm-down stretch.

THE WARM-UP

Cold muscles do not enjoy being stretched. Think of putty or plasticine before you have warmed it in your hands prior to use; if you tried to stretch it in its cold state it would simply tear. Warming-up is essential for three main reasons:

○ The body functions better when warm, enabling the muscles to become more pliable.

○ The warm-up helps you focus and prepare mentally for your workout. It, hopefully, puts you in the mood.

○ Joint mobilisation. Getting your joints loosened up will get synovial fluid into them, as warming them up makes this essential fluid runny and more capable of greasing any stiff joints.

Muscles at rest need only 15% of total blood flow, whereas high activity requires 80% of total blood flow as the muscles demand more fuel. The transfer of the supply cannot happen quickly, and so warm-up should be anything from 5 – 15 minutes, according to the individual and the intended level of exertion.

The activity should be continuous, rhythmic and, ideally, specific or relative to the workout ahead. Always ensure you wear adequate clothing to stay warm; you can always shed your outer layers when you grow warmer.

To stretch or not to stretch before exercise? The debate rages; the argument revolves around the fact that stretching can leave the muscles in a state that makes exercise more difficult, in complete contradiction to the assumed logic that it makes exercise easier.

For years we were told the importance of a short pre-exercise stretch after warm-up and joint mobilisation, taking 6-10 seconds per body part. The stretch was always performed standing as it was considered that lying down or sitting would allow the body to cool, to the obvious detriment of the warm-up. Suddenly – all change! Fitness gurus seem unable to arrive at a unified agreement on this thorny subject. If you read Christopher M Norris's *The Complete Guide to Stretching* it shows research that stretching reduces 'stiffness' before exercise.

If you read Jay Blahnik's *Full-Body Flexibility* he claims such stretching could be unhelpful; I consider both books to be splendid guides on stretching and flexibility, but am left none the wiser.

So – what course to take? If you, like myself, have been doing a short stretch (total time = one minute, see below), for years and have had no ill-effects or loss of performance, (not that I'd notice much these days), my advice is – carry on regardless.

The stretches performed below can be done every day to help you maintain your flexibility level. This is one area in which the timeless maxim "use it or lose it" applies. If you want to get supple, and stay supple, there is no age at which you should think there is a 'cut-off'; continuing stretching will reduce your chances of stiffness and creaky joints in later life.

SHORT STRETCH AFTER WARM-UP

(See The One Minute Stretch below.)

This stretch should be followed by mobility exercises for shoulders, knees, ankles and neck.

MOBILISATION

This consist of some simple and reasonably effortless moves to get all the joints limber.

○ Ankles – point the toe and describe small circles clockwise and anti-clockwise.

○ Knees – knee bends. Any popping sound effects should die off after the first bend.

○ Hips – circle the hips slowly as if exercising with a hula-hoop.

○ Shoulders – roll shoulders to and fro, then gently circle the arms to and fro.

○ Neck – look over one shoulder, then slowly drop the head forward to scan the floor, lifting the head to look over the other shoulder. Repeat 3-4 times.

WARM-DOWN STRETCH

One point all fitness professionals will agree upon is that the optimal time for stretching is after your workout, when the muscles are blood-enriched, warm and, therefore pliable. It will help to speed your recovery, reduce muscular soreness and begin the process of waste clearance.

After your workout it is essential to warm down. It also helps to clear lactic acid and reduce muscle soreness; anyone who has ever suffered the dreaded DOMS (Delayed Onset Muscle Soreness) will appreciate the wisdom of avoiding this particular form of agony by a warm-down and a good stretch. This is when you can lay down on your mat and hold those stretches, now that your warm muscles and ligaments are in a receptive state.

THE STRETCHES

You can avail yourself of any number of books on flexibility which vary in how much technical information and detailed instruction they provide. I have worked on the basis that for now what you need to know is which muscles to stretch and how to stretch them.

I prefer a system whereby I start at the shoulders and work down, making a return trip to finish off with the neck stretch, which I consider the most important as so many retain stress and tightness here. For this reason I have added extra neck stretches.

You should have warmed up for at least 5 minutes prior to stretching – never stretch cold muscles.

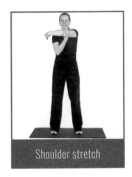

Shoulder stretch

SHOULDER STRETCH

Extend one arm across the chest, then pull it towards you with the other arm.

BACK STRETCH (STANDING)

Used in warm-up stretch. With feet shoulder width apart and slightly bent knees, hold the arms out in front, as if clutching a large beach-ball, while contracting abdominal muscles.

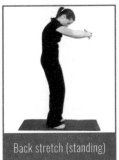

Back stretch (standing)

BACK STRETCH (PRONE)

Lying on a mat, pull your bent legs toward you.

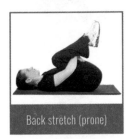

Back stretch (prone)

BACK STRETCH (ANGRY CAT – SPINAL MUSCLES)

While on all fours, haul in the abdominal muscles while rounding the back like a hump-back bridge.

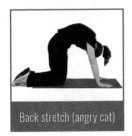

Back stretch (angry cat)

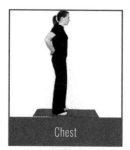

Chest

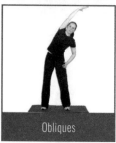

Obliques

CHEST

Hold hands behind your back, raise the arms as you push out the chest.

OBLIQUES

Stand with feet shoulder-width apart, raise one arm then list over to the side.

GLUTES (THE MUSCLES OF THE BACKSIDE)

Raise one leg, then place the other leg across it and pull the lower one toward you.

ADDUCTORS (MUSCLES ON THE INSIDE OF THE LEGS)

While seated place the soles of the feet to touch each other.

HAMSTRINGS (BACK OF UPPER LEG)

Standing version suited to warm up: raise your leg on a bench or similar surface and keeping upper body straight, lean forward.

HAMSTRINGS

Lying version, suited to warm-down: lay on your back, raise your leg in the air and, holding your calf, pull it towards you.

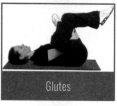

Glutes

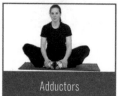

Adductors

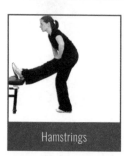

Hamstrings

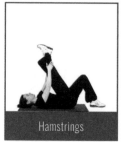

Hamstrings

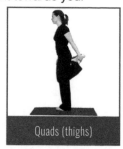

Quads (thighs)

QUADS (THIGHS)

Standing version suited to warm-up: pull lower leg up behind you to touch heel to backside.

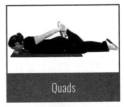

Quads

QUADS

Lying version: lie on front or side, then pull leg back until heel reaches backside.

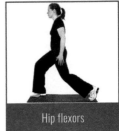

Hip flexors

HIP FLEXORS (PELVIC AREA)

Keep upper body upright as you take a step forward, then lower the hips.

CALF MUSCLES (GASTROCNEMIUS, THE LARGE CALF MUSCLE)

Take a step forward, leaving the heel of the rear foot firmly on the floor as you do. If you cannot feel the stretch, move the rear foot further back until you do.

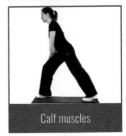

Calf muscles

SOLEUS AND ACHILLES TENDON (LOWER CALF AREA)

Stand with one foot in front of the other with only a small gap between them. Lower your hips as you bend your knees slightly.

TRICEPS (BACK OF UPPER ARM)

Stand with feet shoulder-width apart and take your arms behind your head. Hold the elbow of one arm and gently pull it behind your head.

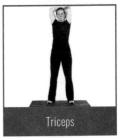

Triceps

NECK MUSCLES

Place your hand on top of your head, then gently ease the head down toward the

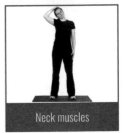

Neck muscles

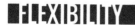

shoulder – do not bring the shoulder up to meet it.

Warmed up and ready for the workout? Take a minute for:

THE ONE MINUTE STRETCH

If you always start at the top and work down there is less chance of missing any muscle group out.

These stretches are held for only 6-8 seconds each. As they usually follow a 5 minute warm-up you are not warm enough to stretch any longer.

Do not hold your breath – breathe naturally.

These are all free-standing stretches, working on the principle you can do them without involving boxes, doorways, mats or any other 'props', so they can be done in a field if necessary.

- ° Neck; look over your shoulder by turning your head slowly to the side. Drop your chin and turn your head to sweep down and across to the opposite shoulder, looking at the ground as you do so. Return to the other shoulder in the same fashion, this will suffice.

- ° Shoulders; raise your left arm straight out in front of you, then, keeping it the same height, take it across your chest until your hand comes in contact with your right shoulder. With your right hand hold the back of the left arm and pull it gently towards the right shoulder. Repeat with the other arm.

- ° Back; with feet shoulder-width apart, bend the knees very slightly. Contract your abdomen while holding your arms out in front of you as if grasping a huge beach ball.

- ° Chest; stand with feet shoulder-width apart with your hands grasped loosely behind your back. Raise your arms behind you and 'lift' your chest as you feel the slight tension applied to it.

- ° Hamstrings; stand with feet fairly close together. Take a large step forward with the left leg. Place the hands flat together against the right (rear) leg. Lift the toe of the left leg until only the heel is on the ground. Keeping the upper body straight lean gently forward, bending the right leg slightly as you do so. Repeat with the other leg.

○ Quads (thigh muscles); stand with feet slightly apart. Keeping your head up, extend your left arm out to the side, to provide balance as you raise your right leg in front of you. Grasp your instep, and pull it gently up behind you. It may be simpler to just raise your leg behind you and locate your instep as it comes up. Personal flexibility will determine how you achieve it.

   ○ If you are a little wobbly when trying this, seek out a solid fixture to hang onto with your free hand, (a companion's shoulder will do nicely). Keep the raised leg very close to the supporting leg as you feel the stretch. Repeat with other leg.

○ Calf Muscles; stand with feet shoulder-width apart, then take a large stride forward with the left leg. Keeping the right leg straight with the heel fully on the ground, bend the left leg and place your hands on the left thigh for support as you bend forward from the waist. Repeat with other leg.

○ Soleus and Achilles tendon; stand with one foot slightly in front of the other, where the toe of the rear foot is slightly behind the heel of the front foot. Hands on hips, let your body weight 'sink' down until you feel the stretch at the lower end of the calf muscle of the rear leg. Keep both heels flat on the floor throughout. Repeat with other leg.

JUST HAVE A STRETCH SESSION

The warm-down stretch can be used as a stand-alone session, just so long as your muscles are warm before you start. Consider taking up Yoga, Tai Chi, Pilates or The Alexander Technique if you want to improve your posture as well as your flexibility. A few years ago these disciplines were considered quite alternative, but many martial artists are now using them to improve strength and flexibility, and they are all, in my opinion, worth trying.

It must be considered that weight training will improve your strength, but not your flexibility, which is an equally important aspect of your well-being; so many people have a good weights workout but neglect to stretch properly afterwards.

Flexibility is the best example of a hackneyed, but nevertheless true, maxim: USE IT – OR LOSE IT.

HELPFUL LITERATURE

○ *Sport Stretch* Michael J Alter (Human Kinetics)

○ *The Complete Guide to Stretching* Christopher Norris (Lyons Press)

○ *Pilates* Michael King (Mitchell Beazley)

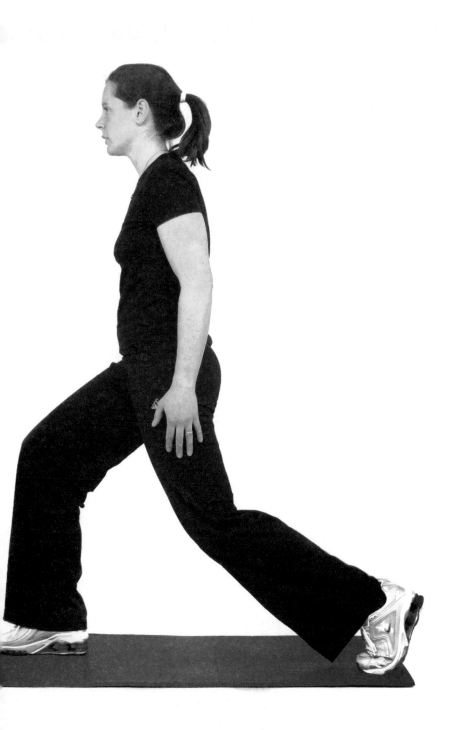

ALTERNATIVE TRAINING

The following advice is for the times, for whatever reason, you simply cannot get any boxing training going. Although the equipment listed below will help maintain fitness, so would shovelling snow, climbing ladders or carrying handfuls of bricks on a building site – as opposed to doing nothing at all.

Specificity is the overriding priority, to get fit for boxing you need to be doing boxing training.

However, if you can't get out into the great outdoors, or the outdoors is not so great due to torrential rain, snow, fog, bone-cutting wind-chill factor or similar dire conditions, then to maintain your fitness level you may have to implement indoor gym training of an alternative nature.

TREADMILL

Running is a specific training tool for boxing, and has been a traditional endurance system for countless years, but sometimes weather conditions or personal circumstances can rule it out. The next best thing to road work is the treadmill. The new types of treadmill can still give you a good running workout (years ago no-one would say that), and they let you know how fast you are going, how far you have run and a (very) approximate calorie count. My verdict is that the treadmill is preferable to not running at all. You might want to consider introducing interval training for improved levels of fitness.

STATIC CYCLE

If for some reason you cannot run e.g. you have a minor calf strain, or knee problems due to pounding the pavement, or there are no facilities for running, a static cycle can help maintain your overall fitness level. Unless stationed in front of a TV, or listening to something on headphones, many would consider static cycling to be somewhat humdrum. Most cycles in the modern gyms have up-to-date machines that give you feedback on speed, distance, heart rate, calories and more. A simple but effective way to get a decent workout from a bike is to work at the following interval training rates*:

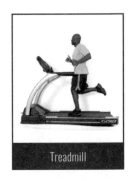

Treadmill

o   3 minute warm-up of easy pedaling.

o   30-60 seconds of flat-out pace.

o   2 minutes easy pedaling for recovery.

o   30-60 seconds flat-out pace.

Continue this pattern, finishing with 5 minutes of easy pedalling to cool down.

* (see also: Tabata Intervals)

ROWING

I must admit I am a fan of rowing machines, and if, for reasons covered in 'Static cycle', you are unable to run, the rowing machine (and my personal favourite, the Concept machines) can give you a good workout.

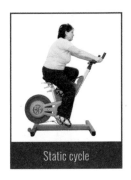

Static cycle

They can:

o   Improve aerobic capacity.

o   Improve muscle tone.

o   Improve stamina.

o   Weight-bearing and impact free (no jarring of joints).

o   If you are using a Concept Rower (most popular model for most gyms), set the pointer to level 6 or 7 (no point in going higher for a cardio

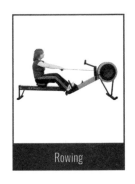

Rowing

workout) and keep the SPM (strokes per minute) over 30.

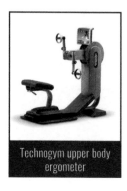

Technogym upper body ergometer

ERGOMETER

Look out for this machine if you train at one of the larger gyms. It is a boon to anybody involved in boxing training, and, out of any of the alternative training equipment listed here, it is probably the most specific for your needs. Evander Holyfield included it in his training programme on the advice of his personal conditioning coach in order to improve upper body strength. If you have managed to get a good cardiovascular workout for your legs on the static cycle, you can do the same for your upper body on the 'Upper Body Ergometer', which will work your abs, back, shoulders and arms. It is primarily designed for upper body strength and conditioning.

It has been described as an 'upper body bicycle'. You simply sit down and turn the handles against a resistance setting. There is also a standing version, which simply means the machine is the same, except the seat has been removed.

On your first efforts on the machine, if it seems like hard going, start with 10 minute sessions on level 5, then build up in increments of 2 or 3 additional minutes on each session. Once you become accustomed to working for longer periods, you can opt for interval training with a 2 or 3 minute easy, 1 minute hard, pattern for 30-45 minutes.

ALTERNATIVE TRAINING
TABATA INTERVALS

I knew of Tabata Interval Training but never really associated it with boxing fitness, and it was not until I read in an article that Manny Pacquiao incorporated it into his training that I took a greater interest.

At the present time Tabata Intervals are growing in use ('popularity' might not be the appropriate term), in just about every sport, and can be used as part of your boxing training. A warning, however, to proceed carefully – this is a very hard form of training.

The Tabata Protocol, or High Intensity Interval Training (HIIT), was developed by the head coach of the Japanese Olympic speed skating team, and took the name of Dr Izumi Tabata, whose team at The National Institute of Fitness and Sport in Tokyo provided the research.

The very term 'Olympic' informs us straight off that this is going to be training aimed primarily at professional or elite athletes, but anybody with a good level of fitness can still benefit from tabata intervals.

When used in boxing, tabatas should be as functional as possible. The patterns of intervals is set whereby the anaerobic work period is double that of the aerobic rest period. This is similar to the work rate in sparring; it is also close to replicating the type of energy level used in a hard sparring session.

It is claimed that 4 minutes of tabatas is as effective as 45 minutes of normal cardio training and can actually play a more effective role in fat reduction.

Tabatas can be successful in deferring the period at which exhaustion is reached, by the way in which they relentlessly push both the mind and body.

Dr. Tabata's team discovered that athletes who used the routine 5 days a week for 6 weeks improved their maximum aerobic capacity by 14% and their anaerobic capacity by 28%, which is highly impressive.

The example shown is that used by elite and professional athletes, and unless you are above average fitness it is best to use one of the easier options shown later in the chapter.

The standard Tabata Interval is to work for 20 seconds (flat out) and rest for 10 seconds (slow recovery rate), which should be repeated 8 times. Before starting it is advisable to warm up for 5 minutes, and to cool down for the same time after the workout. An accurate timer is essential.

SUMMARY OF TIME ALLOCATION;

- ° 5 minute warm up

- ° 4 minutes of intervals (20 seconds + 10 seconds x 8)

- ° 5 minute cool down

- ° Total = 14 minutes

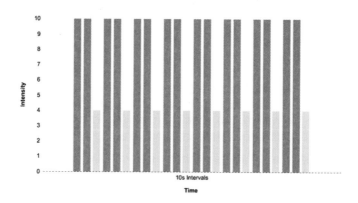

For anybody who wants to try this system I would advise them to start with a modified ratio of work/rest periods. Where the above example shows a negative 'activity to rest' ratio of 2:1, I would modify this to a more realistic 2:2 or 1:3. A beginner who is just starting to get fit should consider a rate whereby they work very hard (not necessarily flat out) for 20 seconds and rest, working at a slow recovery rate, of 60 seconds, and only decrease the rest period once they are much fitter.

The exercises suggested in much of the literature on tabatas states they be used in running/sprinting and cycling, or standing exercises such as squats or burpees*. To make them more specific for boxing training I would suggest the following:

° Skipping.

° Hitting the punchbag (more effective if the bag is held by a partner in the *work phase)*.

° Working on focus pads or a wall pad (straight punches only).

° Roadwork (during a training run).

Tabatas have been described as "4 minutes of pain for great gain", but I will leave you to be the judge of that if you want to try them.

* For Squats and Burpees, see chapter on "Calisthenics".

CIRCUIT TRAINING

You may have done circuit training before, possibly at school, at a gym, or as part of training for football, rugby (or similar sports which require a combination of strength and stamina). It usually consists of several exercise stations set around a hall, gym space or a field to which you progress and then work out for either the allotted time or number of repetitions. Doing it at home will be slightly different (unless you inhabit a cavernous mansion/loft etc.). For those training in the box room, shed garage, or wherever else you have chosen, you will be doing it in the confines of that space, merely picking up or putting down different exercise apparatus. The beauty of circuit training is its flexibility to be adapted to specific needs for individual fitness or training demands. Circuit training is popular because the exercise or equipment is constantly changing which brings an element of freshness to the workout. It is unpopular with some coaches as they consider it a 'shotgun' approach to fitness – if you do enough different exercises you are almost bound to hit a lot of targets, in this case muscle groups; they feel it denigrates technique and is too hard to supervise effectively if the class is large.

Unless you are taking a class and somebody is keeping the tempo by barking out instructions, you can feel free to go at your own pace; I would suggest working 30-40 seconds or 10-20 repetitions at each 'station'.

The type of boxing-functional circuit I have provided in this section is intended purely as an example; you can modify it however you feel to fulfil your personal aims, or simply make your own circuit up, composed of stations you feel best match your needs.

Rather than participants taking an extended rest period (a short rest is fine if the effort is strenuous) I prefer a weight-bearing exercise e.g. squats to be followed by an aerobic exercise e.g. skipping, shadow boxing or jogging on the spot, to prevent tightening up.

° Keep water handy – sip as you go.

○ Have your rope, gloves, timer, weights (if used) etc. handily placed before you start. Saves interrupting your workout to conduct a search.

THE FOLLOWING IS CRUCIAL IN ORDER TO GET YOUR HEART RATE UP AND PREPARE YOU FOR THE CIRCUIT.

WARM-UP

5 minutes of skipping and/or shadow boxing, or a combination of both.

MOBILITY

The mobilisation stage is important; this is where you need to get some synovial fluid (the juice that oils our joints) into your joints.

○ Neck; look over your shoulder, drop your chin to gaze at the ground as you slowly turn to look over the other shoulder.

○ Shoulders; slowly rotate your arms forward and back a few times.

○ Knees; Support your upper body as you raise the knee to form a right angle behind you. Perform in a slow flowing manner for several repetitions.

○ Ankles; slowly rotate your ankle in circles three or four times clockwise and anti-clockwise. Point the toe then bring the toe up toward the shin in an up and down motion.

○ Wrists; slowly rotate your wrist in circles and follow by shaking the fingers as if flicking water off them.

STRETCH

Short stretch; see section on "Stretching – the one minute stretch".

SAMPLE CIRCUITS

There are 2 usual modes of circuit:

○ Circular; the class, or just an individual, works around a circle of exercises going from station to station.

○ Linear; work up and down a straight line, then return to the start to repeat the exercises.

THE 'CONFINED TO QUARTERS' CIRCUIT

Anybody who fancies circuit training at home will have to be content with working in as much space as the room, garage or similar will allow, often in one place, but a versatile circuit is achievable with a little creativity – simply keep all required equipment within reach.

NOTES

○ If you have only one punch bag then use that solely for the 'punching' stations.

○ Insert or substitute any exercises that you feel will be beneficial to your training.

○ Use weights where required if you want to.

○ Don't stick with the same circuit for too long, change it frequently to avoid staleness or reaching a plateau.

○ If training at home – why not put some inspirational music on?

Circuit training is not rigid, and you can be a flexible as you like. Only space and equipment can limit your circuit.

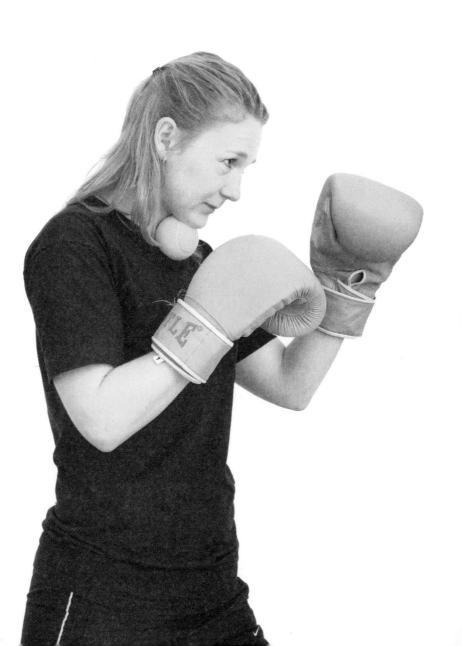

12 STATION LINEAR CIRCUIT | SUGGESTED

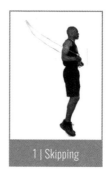

1 | Skipping

1

SKIPPING

Slow and steady

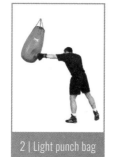

2 | Light punch bag

2

LIGHT PUNCH BAG

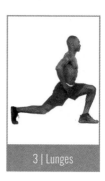

3 | Lunges

3

LUNGES

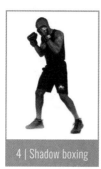

4 | Shadow boxing

4

'HEAVY HANDS' SHADOW BOXING

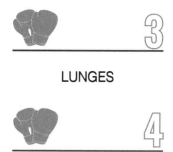

5 | Press-ups

5

PRESS-UPS

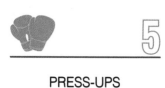

6

STEP-UPS

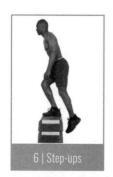

6 | Step-ups

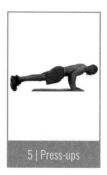
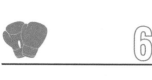

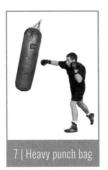

7 | Heavy punch bag

7

HEAVY PUNCH BAG

8

SKIPPING

Fast, running in place

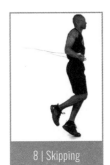

8 | Skipping

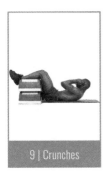

9 | Crunches

9

CRUNCHES

10

SQUATS

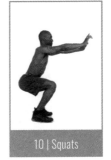

10 | Squats

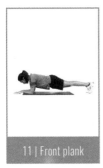

11 | Front plank

11

FRONT PLANK

12

FLOOR-TO-CEILING BALL

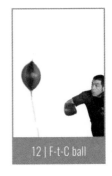

12 | F-t-C ball

EQUIPMENT

PRICE

For many of the items described I have quoted an approximate price, I must point out that this was the retail price as of 2017.

For your specific boxing training needs, there are some obvious requirements you will need straight away, and there are other items you can add as you progress. I have also listed some training equipment which may come in handy. I have no shares or vested interest in Ampro, but they have been making boxing equipment since the 1950s, and it is usually good quality, and, unlike some other boxing manufacturers they do not have a 'fashion' marketing arm.

BAG MITTS

An essential requirement. Always go for good quality leather ones; the vinyl type tends to wear out quickly, offer less protection and split frequently, whereas leather wears well and lets the hands 'breathe'. From this information, you may gather I am not a fan of vinyl gloves.

Make sure you have a little room in your new gloves, for two main reasons:

○ Your hands will become hot if you wear the gloves for a long session, and they will expand slightly. Snug-fitting gloves may prove uncomfortable.

○ You will probably need to wrap your hands, especially if you work on the heavy bag, so leave adequate room for the wraps.

Good quality gloves come in small, medium and large, so you should find a good fit. Even top of the range leather gloves, after extensive use, can begin to smell like a cat that expired several weeks ago. The good news is that this can be easily rectified with treatment by a bacterial surface cleaner, using Dettol or any of the main supermarket anti-bacterial cleaners, which are equally remedial. One squirt into the glove on a regular basis should remove the most pungent odours (works on training shoes as well).

Try to have your own gloves. Some gyms have a 'lucky dip' box full of unloved gloves their owners have long ago abandoned. Unfortunately gloves from this sad and sorry selection tend to leave your hands with a fetid fragrance no soap known to mankind can neutralise for days. The best move is get your own gloves if you intend to train regularly on bags and pads, then reel back the years to your schooldays and write your name or initials on them boldly with a permanent marker, in readiness for those occasions that you depart the gym tired and confused by your exertions and leave them behind. Phoning to report them missing, with the only available description being "they are red", will not be a great help to anybody seeking them, especially if the 'lost and forsaken' box is overflowing with red gloves.

If you find you are having problems with the thumb of your gloves (for some odd reason many manufacturers invariably endow every glove with 'large' size on the thumb), one solution may be a pair of 'thumbless' gloves, or simply prune the thumb of your own gloves with scissors.

Whichever solution you decide upon, strive to ensure your thumb is 'tucked in'.

If you have delicate or vulnerable hands, or are concerned because your hands are vital to your profession, e.g. concert pianist, snooker professional or hairdresser (I've experienced this

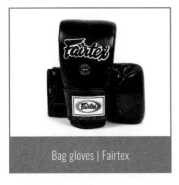

Bag gloves | Fairtex

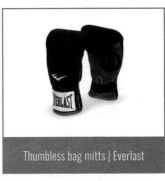

Thumbless bag mitts | Everlast

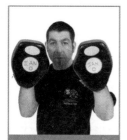

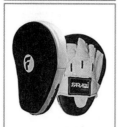

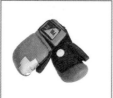

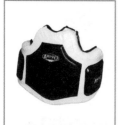

twice), or if your hands are arthritic, I would advise wearing sparring gloves, either 12, 14 or 16oz, to give your hands additional padding to protect them.

A final endorsement of good leather gloves: my archaic Lonsdales are still giving reasonable service (pictured). I bought these what seems like around the time of the fall of Rome. I'd get rid of them but I'm frightened of hurting their feelings…

FOCUS PADS | HOOK & JAB PADS

If you are going to buy your own pads, as with gloves, I advocate getting good leather ones. The vinyl variety are invariably sub-standard, and the canvas variety have as much 'feedback' as a stale bread pudding. Pads may be flat or curved: try to use both at the gym before you come to your decision. I have a pair of each and like them equally. Years ago pads came with buckles and straps, which were fussy and time-consuming, but these have been rapidly replaced with the Velcro fastening variety, making them easy to slip on and off. Try to ensure your hand is a comfortably fit in the 'glove' area of the pad, which is why buying from a boxing store is preferable, which will allow you to try before you buy.

As with your gloves, emblazon your name/initials on your pads with a permanent marker, especially if everybody at the gym uses the same brand.

COACHING MITTS | COACHSPAR MITTS

Coaching Mitts are discussed fully in the section on Focus Pads, but they are not suitable for novices, and good leather ones do not come cheap.

As you can be construed from the sad and sorry state of my own coaching mitts they take quite a battering; mine are around fifteen years old and I bought them from Pro-Box for £35.

The curved Fabari pads seen opposite currently retail at around £30.

BODY PROTECTOR

This useful piece of equipment is for experienced coaches and is a great coaching aid, very popular in professional boxing and many martial arts. The coach can wear this and hold focus pads to enable both head and body shots, and a combination of both. The Ampro model shown below contains a gel padding and retails at around £88.

TIMERS

If you want to work out, or train somebody for a specified period, then you need to know when that 2 or 3 minute round is over. Wearing a watch while holding focus pads, or boxing mitts, is impractical, and glancing up at gym clock at a crucial juncture may prove painful, so use a timer. If the surrounding environment is not too noisy you may be able to use the timer on a stopwatch on a sports watch, digital phone, iPhone or iPad.

Louder and cheaper is a kitchen timer with an audible alarm.

The Salter has a decently audible alarm. Not too 'gym robust', as some mastodon managed to snap the little stand off the back of mine.

THE EVERLAST PERSONAL ROUND TIMER

This is a neat idea. Select 2 or 3 minute rounds: rest times are

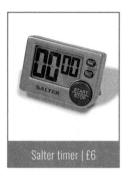

Salter timer | £6

30 or 60 seconds. Each round starts with an authentic ringside bell, but the main problem is there is no volume control. Great if you are training alone in your home or garage – it can be clipped to your waistband or stand-alone – but the alarm is not particularly loud. They can be worn on the arm or wrist. These cost around £25, currently available on eBay UK.

Bell, or vibrating buzzer? You choose.

GYMBOSS TIMER

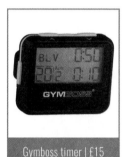

Gymboss timer | £15

Relatively inexpensive, but highly reliable, and very popular with many gyms and trainers, are the Gymboss Timers. Versatile time intervals, large memory, and they can either beep or vibrate. The size of a pager and rubberised for protection. The 'Max Black' (priced at £19.50) version has slightly more features, but the standard version, available in silver, black, pink or green is perfect for personal use, and retails at £15.

There is a Gymboss armband and a wristband, both available at around £3.

BOXING TIME CLOCK

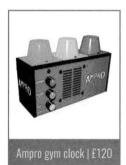

Ampro gym clock | £120

Usually these are only found at the gym, and work off a 240 volt supply. Having one at home can be regarded as possibly luxurious, as they are, at time of going to press, £120. The model shown left has light indicators and a loud bell sound to announce the end of a round. They offer 2 or 3 minute rounds and 30 or 60 second intervals. Expensive but solidly built and robust. Possibly overkill for just training in the garage.

HANDWRAPS

As mentioned earlier, handwraps will protect your hands and wrist and lessen any possible abrasion from your gloves.

The most user-friendly variety is elasticated with Velcro fastening, which stops them unravelling, unlike the plain linen variety. Give your wraps a frequent wash with a little fabric softener added and they will last for years; they are invariably soaked in perspiration after use, and if you consistently forgo washing them they may just slither away on their own – keep them clean.

Should you find your handwraps are incredibly long (many are, as 15' long wraps suit the big-handed type), put them on and work out how much material you have found to be surplus once you have wrapped your hands to your satisfaction. Cut that exact amount from the middle of the wrap, and sew the ends back together – it doesn't matter how good or bad your sewing skill is – nobody is going to see it, and it merely needs to hold together. Your wraps are now 'tailor-made'. The shorter versions are around 8 feet long.

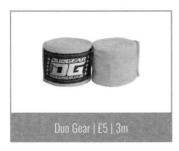

Duo Gear | £5 | 3m

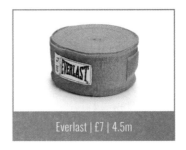

Everlast | £7 | 4.5m

FOOTWEAR

Some people love wearing boxing or wrestling boots (slightly shorter in the leg than classic boxing boots). Some are even happy in bare feet, Thai style. I would advise beginners to wear trainers with some support, such as running shoes, cross-trainers, or tennis shoes. If the shoes can 'slide' a little, all the better for your footwork. Double-knot your laces to prevent a loose lace interrupting your workout.

Boxing boots vary in cost. Try to find a store where you can try them on for size and comfort. An online purchase may be more economical, but you cannot try them on online. Boxing boots will give a good grip and assist the sliding aspect of your footwork. Boxing boots come in high or low leg. As with gloves, always go for leather as synthetic material can 'draw' the feet.

Prices start at around £25 and go up to around £200, but you should be able to pick up a decent pair to start out with for around £30-40.

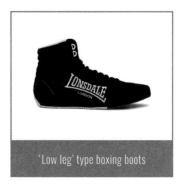

'Low leg' type boxing boots

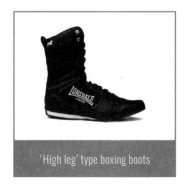

'High leg' type boxing boots

MOUTH GUARD | GUM SHIELD

A gum shield (the old, and most common term) is mandatory if you are going to engage in sparring. Once the gum shield is in your mouth you need to breathe through your nose, as you will need to keep your mouth closed.

Keeping a closed mouth when sparring is vital, as a blow on an open mouth can damage the mandible (jawbone). If the mouth is open the jawbone is isolated, which renders it vulnerable, and can be knocked sideways, causing serious injury, whereas a punch that strikes a closed jaw usually causes the whole head to turn, and the 'clamped' jaw is less likely to be injured. Thus good technique means not only to keep your chin down, in order to avoid any punches on the jaw, but keep your mouth closed in case you sustain such a blow. Breathing while sparring must therefore be done through the nose, (which is approximately 3 times more effective than breathing through the mouth). Wear your new gum shield while shadow boxing to become acquainted to it.

When buying a gum shield I feel that there are three options, best explained as budget, mid-price and expensive. I see them as follows...

BUDGET

These can be picked up for a few pounds. The model shown starts at around £1.50. These are in the D.I.Y range, whereby you drop the gum shield in boiling water for 10 seconds, then fish it out with a spoon or a suitable implement. Next, while it is still warm, pop it into your mouth, clamp your top and bottom teeth together and hold that for another 10 seconds. Remove it from your mouth and drop it into cold water to set.

If your finished effort doesn't seem right – start all over again until you get it right. The slightly more expensive self-fitting type come with a plastic container to keep it in; it is obviously more hygienic to rinse it before and after use and keep it in a clean container between sessions.

MID-PRICE

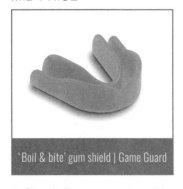

'Boil & bite' gum shield | Game Guard

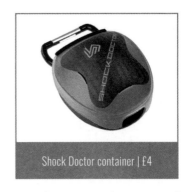

Shock Doctor container | £4

A Shock Doctor version: this company has a massive range of gum shields, and the one shown retails at around £10. It contains gel and provides more padding than the budget range. It claims to provide superior protection, due to its shape, but still needs to be self-moulded with the same procedure as the budget type.

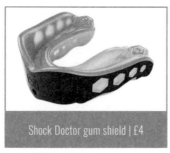

TAILOR MADE

Reach for your credit card as the next version involves your dentist, who will – at a price, take an impression of your teeth (by inserting a wax-filled plate into your mouth), before sending the impression off to be moulded into a perfect-fit gum shield. This procedure will cost, as far as I have discovered to date, somewhere between £100-200. I bought mine from a dentist for £25, at around the time Sinatra was playing The Sands in Vegas – and I had a few more teeth.

You Are the Dentist!

There are online companies who will send you a self-fitting kit from around £20: it is entirely up to individual choice.

- ○ gumshields.com

- ○ mouthguards.opro.com

- ○ funkygums.com

SPARRING GLOVES

Once you have your gum shield snugly in situ, and your hands securely wrapped, you are ready to don your sparring gloves.

These come in 12, 14, 16 and 18oz. They are not just to protect your sparring partner's head and body, but, more realistically, the relatively fragile bones of the hand. The reputable brands make them in all weights; buy the best leather ones you can afford. Treat them properly and they will last for years. Never put them on the floor, as they can pick up bacteria, which, above all, shows a marked lack of respect for your sparring partner. Write your name or initials on them and 'detoxify' them regularly with a squirt of anti-bacterial cleaner, as this should prevent them from forming penicillin between sessions.

The gloves that come with a Velcro fastening are the best bet, as the lace-up variety, which are used in competitions (see Cleto Reyes below), are time-consuming and fiddly, and require help in fastening, unlike the Velcro version.

HEADGUARD

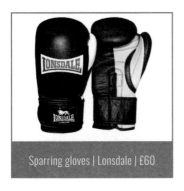

Sparring gloves | Lonsdale | £60

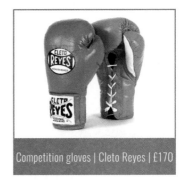

Competition gloves | Cleto Reyes | £170

Formerly compulsory in amateur boxing, and worn by most professionals in sparring, to reduce the risk of facial injury when in training for contests.

The main problem with inexperienced boxers wearing headguards is the danger of becoming a trifle careless, or even reckless, in the belief the headguard affords complete head protection – which it does not. Learning to spar without a headguard teaches you to be more cautious and constantly move your head, as you should. Some headguards can also hinder vision. If you decide to buy one, there are a great many products on the market, and it is best to go for a good quality leather one. There are several types, but I have shown the two most common varieties.

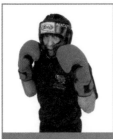

Headguard with cheekbone protection | Fairtex

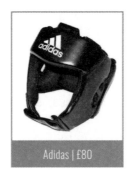

Adidas | £80

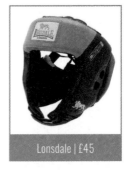

Lonsdale | £45

GROIN GUARD | ATHLETIC CUP

Generally shortened to 'the cup', and highly advisable for serious sparring, for what must be fairly obvious reasons.

There are also heavy-protection types:

° Lonsdale Super Pro (around £45)

° Cleto Reyes (around £90)

Adidas | £16

WOMEN

Again, I see no reason to go into detail here, as I believe a picture is better than ten thousand words. Inserts can also be bought for greater protection.

TRAINING AIDS

PRESS-UP STANDS

I am a big fan of these, particularly as they are both cheap and functional. They allow a greater range of depth to the press-up and, at the same time, take pressure off the wrist.

Combat sports bra | Cool Guard | £22

Press-up/push-up stands sell from anything from £3 to £10.

Mine are made by York, a little worn on the foam, but still giving good service after around 5 years. These are my third pair, as the foam tends to eventually disintegrate through wear and tear.

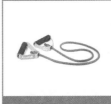

Press-up stands

RESISTANCE BANDS

These are great for home training and extremely versatile. Simply anchor them to a solid fixing and you can perform a huge range of exercises. The bands are colour-coded to ascertain the degree of difficulty of use. The black bands are generally found to be the most resistant. Other colours vary from manufacturer to manufacturer and are usually listed as level 1, level 2 etc. to describe the band's resistance.

Resistance band | Reebok | £10

PULL-UP BAR

Chins, or pull-ups, whichever you prefer, is a challenging exercise targeting the back, shoulders and biceps (according to your grip), but if you don't belong to a gym, can't get to the gym, or your gym does not have a pull-up/chinning bar – then get your own. It is not a long term fixture (or had better not be, in my wife's judgement), just an extending bar that locks into two cups set either side of the doorframe. If you required a bar in order to do inverted rows you only have to set the cups lower in the frame.

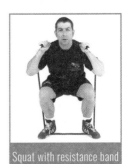

Squat with resistance band

My pull-up bar fits into the doorway of the slightly untidy office at my house, and is strong enough to take my weight (70kg) and as long as the metal cups that take the bar are firmly screwed in place (I used six 4cm

Punching drill using resistance bands

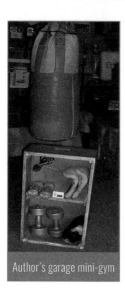

Author's garage mini-gym

screws), it should be fine for somebody of average weight; the manufacturer state it can take support somebody up to around 15 stone in weight – their doorway would need to be a lot stronger than mine, I feel.

Mine is made by York, and I paid around £15 at Argos.

HOME TRAINING MINI-GYM

There was a time when I used to do most of my training in my garage, and I realise that, in the current financial climate, many people are forced to do the same or similar, but this does not mean you can't have a well-structured training session, be it in the garage, shed or spare room.

Shown left, in my garage, in which there is just about enough space to train, is all the kit I need. This consists of a battered second-hand canvas and leather bag, bag mitts, a wooden step-box rescued from a skip it had been relegated to outside the gym, 3kg and 5kg dumbbells, a skipping rope, press-up stands and an Ascot kitchen timer (£1.99 in Aldi). The box is fine for step-ups and doubles as a bench. A discarded length of carpet on the floor is kinder than the concrete below it.

SURPLUS EQUIPMENT

There are certain items that you will *not* be needing when you train, which are as follows;

○ Jewellery. Try to leave your rings, earrings, necklaces, bracelets, bangles etc. at home, and remove any facial piercing to avoid personal injury, loss or damage to the items. If it is going to get in your way, take your watch off, as well.

○ Spectacles and Contact Lenses. No matter how poor your sight is, it should be glaringly obvious that you will not be sparring whilst wearing a pair of glasses. Only wear your contact lenses if you absolutely need them. I lost count of the number of times I had to halt a class in order for everybody to look for a lost contact lens.

○ Baseball Caps. For what seemed an unfathomable reason, some people would occasionally turn up for training wearing a baseball cap. In my experience there were two plausible explanations, which were: firstly, they though it lent an air of panache to their appearance, or secondly, they were conscious of their baldness, as if somebody at a boxing gym would even care. A baseball cap is practical for golfers – 99% of professionals wear one – but in boxing it is a total hindrance, as it limits upward vision and will, invariably, fall off. Whether worn forwards, sideways or backwards – they are totally superfluous; if, for some reason, your head doesn't feel warm enough – wear a knitted cap/bobble hat, or a hooded top until you are warm enough to remove it.

○ Sweat Suits and Bin-liners. It is erroneous to think that by wearing either of these articles you can 'slim down'. You will certainly sweat like the first horse past the post at the Epsom Derby, as he enters the Winner's Enclosure, but as soon as fluid is taken, weight loss is nullified. They also cause you to overheat and become in danger of dehydrating; I have seen people become dizzy and faint after training in them. A professional boxer may resort to a sweat-suit as a short-term measure to make the weight for a fight, but the average trainer should give them a very wide berth.

○ Mobile Phone. Unless you are a medical professional on-call, or an expectant father whose offspring is due at any instant, turn your phone off, or risk the apoplectic rage of your trainer as you breezily answer a call from your mum, boyfriend/girlfriend during a class – such is likely to be the vitriol incurred, I imagine it will only happen once.

○ If you are not in a class and need to use your phone – take it out of earshot of people who are trying to train seriously. Your personal details are not something they are likely to want to be subjected to, and neither is your novel ringtone, and they may forcibly inform you of this fact.

○ To my incredulity, I have witnessed people using a mobile phone while doing sit-ups, also doing one-arm bicep curls, and texting while on the treadmill – I can't help feeling it must detract somewhat from their performance.

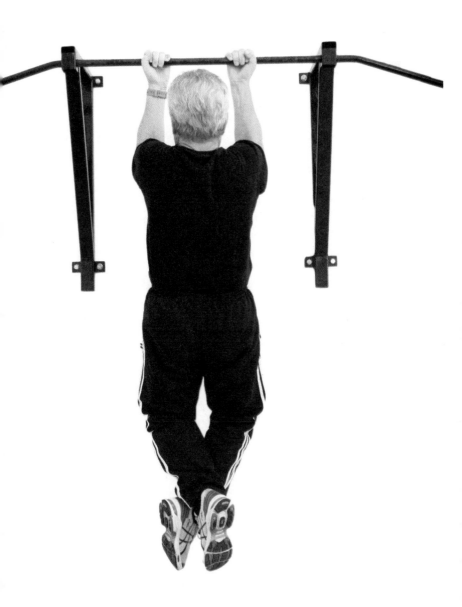

NUTRITION, INJURY & ILLNESS

In this day and age, everybody, even schoolchildren, has a pretty accurate idea about the difference between the kinds of foods that are recommended and encouraged, and those that are unhealthy, or even harmful. We are told to get our "5 a day", cut out fatty foods and, in general, make healthy choices. Whether or not people (even armed with this information) *will* make a healthy choice in the matter is a completely different story. Ironically the unhealthy food, mainly in the form of takeaways and fast food outlets, is chosen because it is regarded as 'cheap' food. In actual fact the cost usually comes not in monetary terms, but in health costs; this stuff can really threaten your state of health, not to mention your waistline. If you are going to start something as strenuous as boxing training then you are going to need more fuel, especially if you have not been involved in sports fitness of this level.

If you are overweight, the good news is that you don't need to starve yourself to lose weight. You are better off *eating* to lose weight. The secret is to eat the right foods and cut out the wrong ones. There is so much information available with regard to the difference between intelligent eating and downright stupid eating. Nobody can really dispute the fact that they don't know the difference; if you intend to get involved in this serious training programme it really is wise to evaluate what kind of intake you will need to fuel your body for your workouts – and then stick to it. We are unlikely to put fuel into our car that may harm the engine, so why would anybody want to put fuel into their body that they know is potentially harmful to their health?

It is fairly obvious that our diet has a significant influence on our fitness performance. A balanced diet, both in quality and quantity before, after, and in some cases, during activity, will greatly benefit performance.

In most cases the balance should be:

  ° 60 – 70% carbohydrate.

○ Approx. 12% protein.

○ The remainder will come from fat, which should not exceed 30%.

When it comes to dropping a few pounds a little research into what you should eat is a good start toward a positive outcome. Expert advice on the subject is not hard to obtain, God only knows how many hours of television time are devoted to it.

The good news is that good foods are in general more filling, whereas junk food tends to leave you feeling unfulfilled, so by improving the quality of your intake you should gradually be satisfied with a smaller volume of food. There is no need, however, to eat food you openly dislike or, worse still, feel you have an allergy to; there is a rich variety of good food available in the shape of fruit, vegetables and starchy food (such as bread, cereal, pasta, potatoes, rice), semi-skimmed milk (skimmed milk always makes me feel as if I'm paying a penance), and lean meats.

If you have the time and the ability (or your partner's ability) try to cook and eat at home, as opposed to getting take-aways or eating out on rich foods. This way you are less likely to add excessive salt or artificial additives of the kind the manufacturers include.

Give your heart a break and cut out unnecessary salt from your diet, especially if there is a history of blood pressure or heart disease in your family history. Read food labels and check out the amount of sodium; high levels can be found in salted nuts, crisps and similar snacks. Choose brands with the lowest sodium levels or make your own soups and cereals. Easy guide cookbooks to whip up healthy concoctions that taste good have never been more abundant.

When training causes sweat loss to become high it is essential to increase your fluid intake to prevent dehydration. A plastic water bottle to always have by you at the gym is one of the smartest investments you can make.

Tip – If you know you are going to have a hard workout – pack a banana (or 2) in your bag.

Anybody involved in competitive boxing should eat within the constraints of a diet that will not jeopardise their weight, to stay within their weight division, as well as being in top fighting shape.

As you are unlikely, at this stage, to be too concerned about making a particular weight, you can just concentrate on eating to train to the best of your capabilities.

The following nutritional advice comes from Victoria Mose (Y.M.C.A. Fitness Industry Training).

HEALTHY EATING

The food we eat plays an essential role in how well we feel and look. Eating a balanced healthy diet can not only keep the body at a healthy weight but also improve the tone and condition of both hair and skin.

This section is designed to give you some basic tips on how to ensure you eat a healthy and balanced diet and how you can incorporate the 5 basic food groups into mealtimes.

The basic food groups are listed in the table opposite.

Tips on how to get the balance right:

- ° Avoid diets – the only diet you should be on is a healthy eating one.

- ° Try to include a range of colours when eating fruit and veg, and eat plenty.

- ° Eat a variety of foods.

- ° Get your portion size right.

- ° Keep alcohol consumption low.

- ° Avoid drinks high in sugar.

- ° Limit the amount of foods high in fat/sugar that you eat.

- ° Eat foods high in starch and fibre.

FOOD GROUP	TYPES OF FOOD	NUTRIENTS	RECOMMENDATIONS
Breads, Cereals, Potatoes	Breads, rice, pasta, oats, noodles etc.	Carbohydrates, (starch) fibre, Vit B, calcium & iron	Try to opt for whole grain bread and pasta. Avoid frying potatoes.
Fruit & Vegetables	Fresh, frozen or canned, beans and pulses can also be included.	Vit C, carotenes, folates, fibre, and some simple carbohydrates	Try to eat fresh as much as possible. Eat a wide range of colours that way you'll get a range of vitamins and minerals.
Milk & Dairy	Milk, cheese, yoghurt, fromage frais.	Calcium, Protein, Vit B12, A & D	Opt for lower fat options. Look at the fat % on a food label a low fat option is something less that 5% fat per 100g. This does not apply to under 5's.
Meat, Fish & Alternatives	Meat, poultry, fish, eggs, nuts, beans pulses.	Iron, protein, Vit B, B12, Zinc, Magnesium	Opt for more white meat a this is lower in fat. Avoid frying and cooking in fat. Try to have fresh meat wherever possible.
Food containing fat: foods and drinks containing sugar	Butter, margarine, cooking oils, salad dressings, cream, chocolate, cakes, puddings etc	Essential fatty acids	Opt for lower fat options but again look at the labels. Avoid hydrogenated fats and too much saturated fat.

- Eat the right amount of food for our gender and age.

- Drink plenty of water.

- Always eat breakfast to kick-start your metabolism.

- Plan your meals – so you don't opt for the quick take away.

- Check food labels – often they say reduced fat but the fat % is still high – general rule is that if it is 5% fat or less per 100g then it is low in fat.

- Want to lose some weight? Have a smaller plate.

PORTION SIZE

A good guide is that a general portion size is the equivalent to your own fist size. Therefore when working out portion sizes you need to measure them approximately to the fist size of the person whose meal it is.

HOW MANY CALORIES DO I NEED?

Calories are the energy currency provided by food. Taking into consideration all you have read so far then you should be able to formulate a balanced diet. The amount of calories needed will depend on the following:

- Your age – older adults generally need less energy (fewer calories) than younger children/adolescents.

- If you are very physically active (average 30mins exercise plus per day) then you'll need more energy than the less active.

- Women generally need less energy than men.

- If you are overweight you'll burn less energy than someone who is a healthy weight.

182 With these things in mind it is very hard to prescribe accurately how many calories a person requires as it can vary from 1,200 to 3,500 calories per day. If you are eating a balanced diet and following the portion size guidelines, then you can't go far wrong. If you are very active, then you may need to increase the amount of fruit/veg and breads and cereals.

HOW DO I GET STARTED?

Keep a food diary for a minimum of 7 days (and no cheating). If you eat a chocolate bar you must write it down. By keeping a diary and writing absolutely everything down this will help you highlight what you are doing right and wrong.

Below is an example of a day from the diary.

DAY 1

BREAKFAST

- ° 2 slices of toast (white bread, butter & jam)
- ° 2 cups of tea (skimmed milk)
- ° 1 small glass of juice

SNACK

- ° 1 KitKat
- ° 1 cup of tea

LUNCH

- ° 1 ham & pickle sandwich (white bread, butter)
- ° 1 bag of crisps
- ° 1 low fat yoghurt
- ° 2 cups of tea

DINNER

- ° 1 frozen pizza

- ° Oven chips

- ° Chocolate ice-cream

- ° 1 glass of water

SNACK

- ° Sweets while watching TV

So analysing the above here are some instant changes that can be made to make this daily intake more balanced and healthy.

CHANGES TO DAY 1

BREAKFAST

Change the bread to whole grain and the spread to low fat, jam on 1 slice or no jam, large glass of juice, 1 cup of tea.

MID MORNING

Fruit and water

LUNCH

Change bread for whole grain, change butter, look at the pickle and select a low sugar salt version, no crisps, replace with fruit or tomatoes/sliced vegetables. 1 cup of tea but also drink some water.

DINNER

Homemade pizza (this is better than take away as take away tend to have lots of oil in the base to keep them hot). Include fresh vegetables and less cheese on the topping. Change the dessert for fresh fruit. Drink of water.

Avoid sweets late in the evening – if you must have something then dried fruit or a small handful of nuts (however these are quite high in calories).

By making the above changes you will increase the whole grain carbohydrate, decrease the fat/sugar, increase the water intake, increase the fruit and vegetable intake and lower the salt and sugar. You can find lots of comprehensive advice about healthy eating on the web. Some useful websites are:

○ www.bda.uk.com

○ www.nhs.uk/change4life

○ www.eatwell.gov.uk.

Eating a balanced diet is essential if you want to change the way you look and feel. Exercise on its own will not do it, as you need the fuel to maintain the exercise. High sugar foods have a fast energy boost effect but they also have a fast to tire effect, so if you are exercising regularly you need a good supply of the whole grain carbohydrates (complex carbs) to be able to keep going.

Good luck with your healthy eating plan and remember it is about changing your lifestyle not going on a 2 week quick fix – quick to undo diet. A slow change over a long period of time is easier to sustain than a rapid weight loss programme – you only have to look at the celebrities that make exercise videos for the new year, most of them have put the weight back on by the following year (with or without the airbrushing!).

WATER

It is generally considered the rule of thumb that mankind can live 3 weeks without food, but only 3-7 days without water. If you are going to train hard then you will need adequate hydration. Unlike a camel you cannot 'load up' with enough fluid to last throughout a strenuous workout: you need to top up at regular intervals. On the other hand, there is no need to guzzle huge amounts of water, as this can affect the body's blood sodium level (hyponatraemia). Up to 8 glasses a day are recommended, but 2 or 3 are still better than none at all, as some hardworking souls do not always get the opportunity to achieve 8 a day. Water should not be ice-cold – room temperature is considered the best.

PRE-TRAINING FOOD

Your basic need is for something that you personally can digest fully, ideally at least 1-2 hours before your workout; it is all very well to advise bananas (which are excellent), if they sit comfortably with your digestion.

If you can digest these, you can try:

○ Fresh fruit.

○ Diluted fruit juice (half and half with water).

○ Bowl of cereal (Weetabix, Shredded Wheat, Cheerios) with semi-skimmed milk).

○ Honey on toast.

○ Peanut butter on toast or crackers.

○ A banana sandwich made with honey or peanut butter (*no butter or margarine*).

○ Smoothie – shop bought, or home-made (see below).

○ Jam sandwich (see "The Flying Scotsman" below).

BANANA & HONEY SMOOTHIE (NEEDS A BLENDER / SMOOTHIE MAKER)

Ingredients

○ 1 ripe banana

○ 1 pint of semi-skimmed milk

- ○ 1 low-fat banana flavoured yoghurt

- ○ 1 dessertspoon-full of honey

- ○ A handful of ice cubes

- ○ 1 scoop of low-fat ice cream (optional)

Blend the banana, cut into chunks, with a small amount of milk. Add the ice cubes and blend them. Add the rest of the ingredients and blend on a high setting. Makes 2-3 good-sized servings.

Drink one serving before exercise, put the rest in the fridge to be consumed after exercise for 'refuelling'.

SPORTS DRINKS VS WATER

Sports drinks claim to refuel more effectively than water. Many recent findings tend to contradict this view.

My take on this is that if you swear that bottle of Lucozade or Gatorade or similar has always been a help, then as long as you don't overdo the fluids I see little harm in it.

I used to try them now and again, but never believed they made a difference, but when I get back from a run I use my own, uncomplicated recipe for refuelling;

- ○ Boil a half litre of water, allow to cool. Add a half a litre of your favourite pure fruit juice, add a pinch of salt. Mix well and refrigerate, or simply drink at room temperature.

THE FLYING SCOTSMAN

Graeme Obree, known as "The Flying Scotsman", is a former world individual pursuit cycling champion, who has twice broken the cycling world hour record. He disdains the use of sports drinks and nutrition supplements. His recipe for sports nutrition is jam sandwiches (on white bread – easier to digest than brown) to provide energy whilst cycling, and for recovery – sardines and broccoli.

Combat and high impact sports can get you into great shape, but you also run the risk of injury, mild or otherwise.

As soon as you feel pain – stop training. If you do not know what is causing the problem, seek the advice of somebody who is likely to know. If your injury is long-term it does not necessarily mean you cannot train at all. Do what you can within the bounds of sound sense and comfort. Leg injuries, according to severity, do not mean you cannot train your upper body, just as a sprained wrist or elbow ligament problem will not prevent leg training.

Do not put off getting a chronic problem examined professionally. If you get no satisfaction with the National Health Service (some do, some don't in my experience), think about consulting a private specialist, preferably on recommendation; this way you may learn how to 'self-help' in the future.

FIRST-AID

Every adult should try to attend a first-aid course, especially if they are a parent. Even without attending a course there are some simple rules to follow when it comes to injury to yourself or a training partner. The very minimum you should familiarise yourself with is "RICE":

- REST
  Stop training immediately.

- ICE
  Get some ice, very cold water or a freeze-spray, applied to the site of the injury as soon as possible, and try to keep it on for 20 minutes every following hour. Do not apply ice directly to the skin – wrap in a cloth/thin towel, to prevent 'ice burn'.

○ COMPRESSION
Strap it up to prevent painful movement and limit swelling. Crepe bandage or 'tubigrip' will suffice.

○ ELEVATION
Raise the injured limb to allow blood to flow back to the heart. If you have limped indoors with a sprained ankle, prop your leg up on the arm of the settee, and pop phone books, catalogues or similar hefty tomes under the legs at the foot of the bed in order to elevate the injury overnight.

If 'RICE' is all you know, then that will be a good start. If, however, the injured person is in agony, or has obviously suffered a major trauma, which could be a fracture, major ligament damage or similar, do not attempt anything – send for an ambulance, and make them comfortable while you wait.

TRAIN SENSIBLY

Don't take unnecessary risks like carrying on when you are in agony. Muscle and ligament damage cannot be "run off"; never ignore your body's signals and try to spot potential trouble and get a diagnosis before it gets worse.

Do not run on icy pavements or on foggy evenings.

Try to always get a decent sleep, and take it a little easier the next day if you didn't get much sleep the night before.

REST & RELAXATION

You should not attempt to train every day. By doing so you are defeating your objective and preventing positive progress. Adaptation, the minimal changes to the body brought about overload, need rest to make improvements. Uninterrupted training and no rest prevents this.

Teach yourself to relax; there are numerous ways and means to educate yourself on this subject. Try books or online sites. No matter how facile some of the suggestions are, it's just possible there may be something useful. Meditation works for some people; don't knock it until you have tried it – Chuck Norris always swore by it, which got my attention.

ILLNESS

There will, inevitably, be times when you fall prey to the odd cold. The general rule of thumb regarding training is;

If it's from the neck up (head cold, sniffles etc.), train lightly.

If it's from the neck down (aching limbs, coughing, wheezing, feeling of lethargy), do not train at all. Wait for the 'all clear' before recommencing.

When returning to training after illness or injury, ease your way back into your fitness regime; you cannot catch up on lost time by overworking.

If friends or training partners tell you that they think you look unwell or off-colour, take notice and proceed carefully: you might be coming down with something. Unsurprisingly, nobody wants to share your illness, and gyms are a prime place to catch something contagious or infectious, so be considerate.

THE RETURN FACTOR

If you got yourself into shape and then succumbed to a bout of the flu, or sprained your ankle, or some other debilitating circumstance, then you must give regular training a miss altogether.

When you come back to training after an extended interval you should not pick up exactly where you left off. The good news is you do not have to go all the way back to where you started – just half way is fine. Take it a little easier than you had been doing prior to your enforced rest, then gradually try to get back to the point where you were before being forced to stop.

INSURANCE

You might want to consider taking out personal insurance. Some gyms have it as a requirement; it is usually as much to cover an unintentional accident to some unfortunate individual, as to yourself personally. If you are self-employed this is well worth investigating.

PAINS & STRAINS

WRIST AND FOREARM STRAIN

The most common pains and strains in boxing novices are usually to the hand, wrist or forearm tendons. This is generally through poor technique in either hitting or holding the pads. If you feel pain in these areas – stop training and use the "RICE" system to start recovery as soon as possible.

After you have got over your injury, is it wise to take advice about your technique from an instructor. The next step is to strengthen the hands and forearms.

It is possible that you are a newcomer to holding focus pads and your forearm muscles are taking on a repetitive challenge they have never previously encountered. As soon as the initial pain subsides, set about strengthening the hand and arm, particularly the forearm.

Get a squeezy/squishy ball, or a foam ball – a squash ball is ok if you don't have a squeezy ball. Simply squeeze the ball until your hand muscles ache, then switch hands. Use it when watching something stultifying on television: it strengthens the hand and forearm muscles.

To build stronger forearm muscles you will need to use a weight; the illustration shows a 3kg dumbbell, but a can of soup, rice pudding etc., will be fine to start with if a dumbbell isn't available. Try doing every other day, take the day off in between for recovery. Shown below are the 'wrist roll' with both Upward roll (undergrip) and Downward roll (overgrip). A combination of them both performed regularly should make a significant improvement to your forearm strength, especially if you gradually move on to a slightly heavier weight when the weight you are using no longer feels heavy.

To do the wrist roll place your forearm on a flat, stable surface, while holding the weight, palm upward for upward roll, palm downward for downward roll. Grip the forearm with your other hand to isolate the wrist.

I should point out that there is only a small amount of movement in each exercise.

Upward Roll

Hold the weight in an undergrip and slowly bring the hand up towards you, so the knuckles face you.

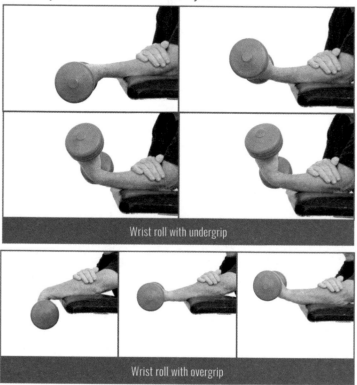

Wrist roll with undergrip

Wrist roll with overgrip

Downward Roll

Holding the weight in an overgrip and slowly bring it upward as far as you can, so the back of the hand faces you.

192 For both exercises start with 3 sets of 10 repetitions.

ACHILLES TENDON AND CALF STRAIN

Boxing means you are going to spend a great deal of time moving around on the balls of your feet, and also putting in some lengthy spells of skipping. Both of these activities place stress on the calf muscles, as does roadwork if you have a tendency to run on your toes. Once again, if it is painful, apply the 'RICE' technique. Once the pain subsides there are, literally, steps you can take to stretch and strengthen your calf muscles. In addition to the calf exercises shown in the chapter on "stretching and flexibility", there are other specific calf stretches you can supplement your recovery with.

The doorstep stretch

Supporting your upper body, allow your heels to overhang the edge of a step, stair or box of similar height. Lean forward and let your heels drop as low as they can go. Hold this for 10-15 seconds.

Seated calf stretch

Take a resistance band, towel or thick skipping rope, and loop it around your raised foot while you are seated. Pull hard as your toes push forward against the resistance.

Shin splints

With this condition, pain is felt at the front of the lower leg, along the shinbone. It often starts out as a nagging ache, which can gradually increase, with activity, into a quite painful and debilitating condition. It may be caused by landing heavily and repeatedly on hard surfaces, poor technique, an awkward movement or ill-fitting unsuitable footwear.

Self-help involves using ice as soon as possible (see home massage below). As soon as pain allows, start stretching by pulling your toes towards you, preferably against resistance for more effect. Sit down and insert your toes under a heavy bench, (or settee), then extend your legs fully until you feel the effect of the action on the injury site. Alternatively, get a friend to stand on your toes, or hold them with his hands, as you recline.

Also try folding your legs underneath you, feet flat against the floor, then sit back on them.

Rest is, unfortunately, vital until all pain subsides. Soldiering on with gritted teeth will only prove detrimental.

NOSEBLEED

When sparring you might just be unlucky enough to sustain a nosebleed. They are unpleasant, but usually only a minor setback – however your training session will almost certainly be over for the evening. They are not uncommon, and it does not always take a particularly heavy blow. Some people get them by merely sneezing, so sometimes a light tap on the nose can cause it.

If you are unlucky enough to get one, or you cause your partner to get one, take the following actions:

º Sit down, lean your head forward and, with thumb and index finger, pinch the fleshy part of the nose, situated just below the bridge of the nose, for 10 minutes.

º Breathe through the mouth but avoid talking or swallowing.

º Release your grip on the nose and check to see if the bleeding has stopped (in which case the blood should have clotted).

º If it starts bleeding again – start the procedure all over again.

º Sit at rest for as long as you can, and, after moving on, do not exert yourself, or blow your nose.

º If the bleeding carries on for longer than 30 minutes, get it checked out at the hospital.

Do not – tip the head back (this is 'old' thinking and blood can run down the throat and cause vomiting).

Do not – jam large amounts of cotton wool up the nostrils to stop the bleeding, as this builds up harmful internal pressure.

Failing that – reach for The St. John Ambulance First Aid Manual. Every gym should have a copy.

PREVENTION OF NOSEBLEEDS

Many boxers, mostly professionals and successful amateurs, undergo cauterization, which is aimed at stopping, or at least reducing nosebleeds. It is not the most pleasant medical procedure, in which the tissue is subjected to a high heat. Some cauterization has been superseded with a process known as electrocoagulation, wherein a high frequency electric current seals the blood vessels in order to inhibit bleeding.

As it sounds, these are serious procedures for serious competitors only. Novices are better off risking a nosebleed.

MASSAGE

Massage is an ancient healing art and can often achieve outstanding results where other healing has failed. It relaxes tired bodies and eases stiff muscles and joints. A session with a professional masseur/masseuse is highly efficacious, but if you need regular massage it can prove expensive. Home massage is an alternative.

In the list of useful literature I have included *Sports & Remedial Massage,* by Mel Cash, and *The Complete Guide to Massage* by Susan Mumford, both of which have a chapter on self-massage, in case you are not in a position where somebody can give you a massage.

Massage oil can be bought ready-made, but it is equally effective, and much cheaper, to make your own. Use almond or grape seed oil as the 'carrier' oil (the bulk liquid), although baby oil or olive oil will suffice, then add the essence of your choice, such as lavender, camomile, peppermint, or any from the enormous range available.

THE MIX

Take a leak-proof plastic bottle – if you take the oil with you, you do not want everything in your bag to reek of essence.

Fill the bottle almost to the neck, about 80% full, then add just 2-3 drips of essence if it is a small, portable bottle; for home use you might want a half-litre bottle, in which case add 7-8 drips of essence. At the time of writing a litre of Grapeseed oil is £3.89 at Tesco, 250 mil of Almond Oil £1.69 at Sainsbury, a bottle of 'lavender essential oil' can be picked up from £3 at most supermarkets or health stores.

All you need to do now is to rub it in; a massage book will tell you the required technique, but if you rub toward the heart until the skin reddens (known as hyperaemia), that will be a good start. Apply the oil to warm hands, and then to the body – never apply oil directly to the body.

ICE MASSAGE

You can use this handy little advice anywhere on the body, but it is extremely effective for the forearm (tennis elbow or golfer's elbow – pad holding can give you either), and for strains in the calf muscles.

○ Take a Styrofoam cup (one of those that break into thousands of miniscule white balls when crushed), and fill to the brim with cold water.

○ Place the container in the freezer. I set it into a second cup to give it additional strength, as these cups are flimsy.

○ At the first onset of a mildly strained muscle take the container and cut around the brim with a sharp knife to remove the top half an inch.

○ Massage the hard protruding dome of ice around the injured site until the ice softens and becomes unusable.

○ Time over small areas should be around 5-10 minutes.

◦   Replace cup in freezer.

Repeat every time you need it, until it becomes too small to be practical. For this reason, keep 2 or 3 in the freezer. I have seen these cups online selling for 70p (25 x 7 oz. cups).

FOAM ROLLERS

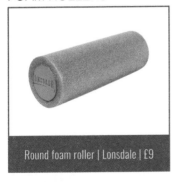

Round foam roller | Lonsdale | £9

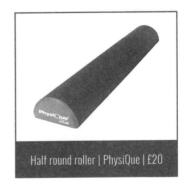

Half round roller | PhysiQue | £20

These rollers, in the shapes depicted here, generally come in two different lengths – 45cm (18") or 90cm (36") – and are either round (left) or half-round, also referred to as 'D' shape or half round (right).

They are inexpensive. The 3' foam roller I bought is made by '66 Fit Elite' and cost £15.

The rollers can be used for core exercises and balance exercises, and are common in yoga and pilates classes. Apart from the balance issue I feel their functionality in this book is with massage more so than any foam roller exercise, as the boxing exercise section covers more specific training, but I think they are a great addition to remedial fitness.

If your muscles feel sore after training then it is worth spending a brief time using a foam roller; it is also a good idea to use one regularly for maintenance reasons, ensuring good tone in your muscles.

The foam roller works for 3 main reasons:

◦   It stretches muscles and tendons.

○ It breaks down adhesions (scar tissue).

○ It softens and lengthens the muscle.

The third effect, softening and lengthening, comes into effect as you use the roller in the manner of a huge, foam rolling pin, ironing and squeezing out knots in your muscles.

The roller works on a principal referred to as 'self-myofascial release' (SMFR), where the term 'myo-' is a prefix for anything related to muscle, and 'fascia' is the sheath containing muscle, tendon and bone; it is probably more easily expressed as 'self-massage'.

Use your bodyweight to locate the sore, or tender, area, then apply pressure as you gently roll the affected area to and fro over the roller.

The troublesome area is known as the trigger point, and once you have located it, if you are employing the use of a high density foam roller which gives a firmer and more intense massage, then you should have little difficulty in locating it. Focus your attention in that small area. Although this procedure, lingering on the tender spot as you concentrate your weight onto the roller, can be moderately painful, consider you are being cruel to be kind to your muscles, relieving their long-term soreness.

FOOT MASSAGE

I have found that although the foam roller is excellent for body massage, it is limited if you have aching feet following your training. This is usually because of rebounding exercises on fallen arches (our arches tend to slowly head south as we age).

If this is the case, take a golf ball, place on the floor and gently roll to and fro to let the dimples on the ball do the massage on your bare foot, (a little massage oil or talc can assist by eliminating friction). Anybody who has suffered the dreaded 'plantar fasciitis', also known as 'policeman's heel' should be acquainted with this helpful procedure.

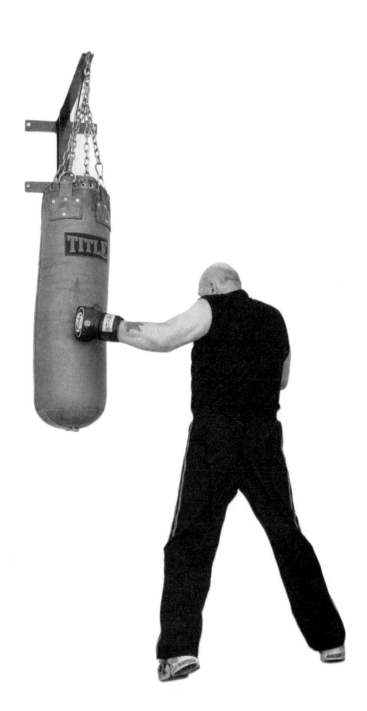

TRAINING FOR SENIORS
THE AGE FACTOR

If you are somewhat mature but reasonably fit, with no debilitating injuries and full medical clearance, and are prepared to take a patient, sensible view about your fitness aspirations, there is a great deal of boxing fitness you can participate in and derive benefit from.

A once-a-week session of light skipping, punching bags and/ or pads, some weight training, jogging or running should not over-extend seniors, particularly those with a history of sporting involvement.

Consider the vast number of runners aged 60 and 70-plus who canter through the London Marathon, and myriad others in Europe and the U.S..

Flexibility training is a must for the mature trainer; the term "use it or lose it" is most apt in this respect. Furthermore, countless tests conducted by universities in the U.S. show that both men and women can make impressive strength gains through resistance training even into their 80s and 90s.

Moderation is the key; work comfortably within your limits at first, and make sure you are ready before you attempt something challenging.

Unfortunately, injury comes easily to the senior trainer, and seems to take forever to clear up.

Never write yourself off. After all, this kind of training should give you renewed confidence and self-esteem. Most people find they enjoy beating the daylights out of a punch bag – it certainly helps to relieve their stress.

Getting into a structured pattern of boxing exercise will improve:

○ Stamina.

○ Muscular Strength.

○ Flexibility and Suppleness.

○ Balance and Co-ordination.

I regard all the above to be vital ingredients when we are getting on in life.

Simply modify the training levels and times to suit your own needs and situation.

Never, at any time, worry about what other people might be thinking, as it is of no matter. Fortunately, I have rarely come across ageism when it comes to this kind of training. Younger onlookers, at least those with a modicum of intelligence, will in all probability admire you for signing up to this level of training, hoping they can emulate you when they reach your age.

IT'S IN THE BAG
PACKING FOR THE GYM

First, get the largest, sturdiest bag you can carry so you are well prepared with all your kit on board.

Don't forget:

- Flip-flops: avoid foot infections, particularly verrucas – they are harder to get rid of than a tattoo.

- Plastic bag (a carrier bag will do) to keep your wet stuff away from the items you need to keep dry, and to avoid getting that 'swimming bath' odour in your bag.

- Water bottle: stay hydrated, get a fair-sized one and sip as you train, tap water should be fine, avoid 'ice' water.

- Skipping rope: if you intend to skip at the gym, take your own rope, as theirs may all be in use, or too long/short for you.

- Warm-up gear: if the gym tends to be on the cool side, i.e. no heating, or somebody has been over-zealous with the air conditioning, throw in a thick sweatshirt, possibly with a hood, which you can peel off when you are warm. If it is cold, pack a woolly hat and track bottoms. Avoid starting your exercise with cold muscles.

- Boxing tape/surgical tape: needed to cover the laces if you have lace-up sparring gloves and handy for various repairs to kit.

- Petroleum jelly (Vaseline): smear this lightly over the eyebrows if you have the problem of sweat running into your eyes and causing them to sting and impairing your vision. Also good for protection against chafing and friction from clothing, especially new garments.

IN THE WASHBAG

Apart from shower gel, toiletries etc., include these inexpensive but very useful accessories.

- Vaseline (reasons given above).

- Small packet of plasters.

- Small pair of nail scissors – not just for nails, more for general purpose, and some safety pins for any emergency repairs.

- Small plastic bottle of massage oil (see 'Massage' in chapter on "Illness and Injury") if you think you will need to apply it before or after your workout.

- Packet of clean tissues and medi-wipes.

- Arnica cream; for bruises (some believe in it, some don't, I still do).

GOOD TO KNOW
USEFUL LITERATURE

- The Lonsdale Training Manual
  David James (Robson Books)

- Sports Nutrition Guidebook
  Nancy Clarke (Human Kinetics)

- The Complete Guide to Sports Nutrition
  Anita Bean (A & C. Black)

- The Complete Guide to Strength Training
  Anita Bean (A & C. Black)

- The Complete Guide to Core Stability
  Matt Lawrence (A & C. Black)

- Strong to the Core
  Lisa Westlake (Aurum Press)

- Core Performance Essentials
  Mark Verstegen (Rodale)

- Core Training Anatomy
  Frederic Delavier (Human Kinetics)

- Strength Training Anatomy
  Frederic Delavier (Human Kinetics)

- Fitness and Health
  Brian Sharkey (Human Kinetics)

- The Complete Guide to Functional Training
  Allan Collins (Bloomsbury)

- The Complete Guide to Kettlebell Training
  Allan Collins (Bloomsbury)

- Running: Getting Started
  Jeff Galloway (Meyer & Meyer)

- Strength Band Training
  Page & Ellen Becker (Human Kinetics)

- The Complete Guide to Stretching
  Christopher Norris (A & C. Black)

- Sport Stretch
  Michael J Alter (Human Kinetics)

- Stretching
  Bob Anderson (Shelter Books)

- Full-Body Flexibility
  Jay Blahnik (Human Kinetics)

- Anatomy of Exercise
  Pat Manocchia (A & C. Black)

- Functional Training for Sports
  Mike Boyle (Human Kinetics)

- Athletic Body in Balance
  Gray Cook (Human Kinetics)

- Box Like the Pros
  Joe Frazier & William Dettloff (Collins)

- Sparring
  Bob Breen (Bob Breen Academy)

- Sports Injuries
  Vivian Grisogono (Lotus Publishing)

- Jump Rope Training
  Buddy Lee (Human Kinetics)

- The Official British Army Fitness Guide
  Sam Murphy (Guardian Books)

- First Aid Manual
  St John's Ambulance (Dorling Kindersley)

- Sports and Remedial Massage Therapy
  Mel Cash (Ebury Press)

- Foam Roller Workbook
  Dr. Karl Knopf (Ulysses Press)

- The Concise Book of Muscles
  Chris Jarney (Lotus Publishing)

GOOD TO KNOW
MODELS & AUTHOR

BOXING FITNESS NEW EDITION MODELS

- Dave Birkett
- Owen Ogbourne
- Victoria Mose
- Shereen Rowe
- Wayne Rowlands
- Stephanie De Howes
- Corey Donoghue
- Howard Newton
- David Thorp
- Samantha Russell
- Tanya Rahman
- Oliver Sebe
- Lara Venables
- Steve Wright (sans 'tache)
- Sally Bladon
- Al Livingstone

THE AUTHOR | IAN OLIVER

Ian Oliver is the former (now retired) boxing coach of The Bob Breen Academy of Martial Arts of Hoxton, East London.

He has made regular contributions to Men's Fitness, Men's Health and Arena Magazine, and is the author of 'Punch Your Way to Fitness', 'Fifty Plus Fitness' and 'Toughen Up', and the DVD 'Boxing Fitness'.

He was born in Hackney, East London and now resides in Chelmsford.